MW01013829

Appleton & Lange's Review of
MAMMOGRAPHY

Olive Peart, MS, RT(R)(M)
Clinical Instructor
Program in Radiography
The Stamford Hospital
Stamford, Connecticut

Appleton & Lange Reviews/McGraw-Hill
Medical Publishing Division

New York   Chicago   San Francisco   Lisbon   London   Madrid   Mexico City
New Delhi   San Juan   Seoul   Singapore   Sydney   Toronto

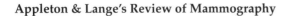

McGraw-Hill

*A Division of The **McGraw·Hill** Companies*

Notice

Medicine is an ever-changing science. As new research and clinical experience broaden our knowledge, changes in treatment and drug therapy are required. The authors and the publisher of this work have checked with sources believed to be reliable in their efforts to provide information that is complete and generally in accord with the standards accepted at the time of publication. However, in view of the possibility of human error or changes in medical sciences, neither the authors nor the publisher nor any other party who has been involved in the preparation or publication of this work warrants that the information contained herein is in every respect accurate or complete, and they disclaim all responsibility for any errors or omissions or for the results obtained from use of the information contained in this work. Readers are encouraged to confirm the information contained herein with other sources. For example and in particular, readers are advised to check the product information sheet included in the package of each drug they plan to administer to be certain that the information contained in this work is accurate and that changes have not been made in the recommended dose or in the contraindications for administration. This recommendation is of particular importance in connection with new or infrequently used drugs.

This book was set in Palatino by Rainbow Graphics.
The editors were Trish Casey and Catherine A. Johnson.
The production supervisor was Lisa Mendez.
The indexer was Susan Hunter, Andover Publishing Services.
Von Hoffman Graphics was printer and binder.

This book was printed on acid-free paper.

Library of Congress Cataloging-in-Publication Data

Peart, O. J. (Olive J.)
Appleton & Lange's review of mammography / Olive Peart.—1st ed.
    p. ; cm.
  Includes bibliographical references.
  ISBN 0-07-137828-6 (alk. paper)
    1. Breast—Radiology—Examinations, questions, etc. 2.
Breast—Cancer—Diagnosis—Examinations, questions, etc. 3.
Breast—Imaging—Examinations, questions, etc. 4. Medical screening—Examinations, questions, etc. I. Title: Appleton and Lange's review of mammography. II. Title: Review of mammography. III. Title.
  [DNLM: 1. Mammography—Examination Questions. WP 18.2 P362a 2002]
RG493.5.R33.P435 2002
616.99′44907572′076—dc21   2002016683

Contents

Preface v

Acknowledgments vii

Bibliography ix

1. Patient Education and Assessment 1

   Summary of Important Points 1
   Questions 4
   Answers and Explanations 8

2. Instrumentation and Quality Assurance 13

   Summary of Important Points 13
   Questions 18
   Answers and Explanations 24

3. Anatomy, Physiology, and Pathology of the Breast 35

   Summary of Important Points 35
   Questions 39
   Answers and Explanations 44

4. Mammographic Technique and Image Evaluation 49

   Summary of Important Points 49
   Questions 51
   Answers and Explanations 56

5. Positioning and Interventional Procedures 61

   Summary of Important Points 61
   Questions 68
   Answers and Explanations 75

6. Practice Test 1 . . . . **83**

Questions *83*
Answers and Explanations *97*

7. Practice Test 2 . . . . **111**

Questions *111*
Answers and Explanations *124*

Index **141**

Preface

This book is a review and self-assessment manual for radiologic technologists, its purpose being to help technologists who are considering the Advanced Level Examination in mammography. The book follows the content category guidelines as specified in the examinee handbook published by the American Registry of Radiologic Technologists (ARRT).

The ARRT does not review, evaluate, or endorse publications. Permission to reproduce ARRT copyrighted material within this publication should not be construed as an endorsement of the publication by the ARRT.

The first five chapters review the content category guidelines: (1) Patient Education and Assessment, (2) Instrumentation and Quality Assurance, (3) Anatomy, Physiology and Pathology of the Breast, (4) Mammographic Technique and Image Evaluation, (5) Positioning and Interventional Procedures (© 2002 by The American Registry of Radiologic Technologists). Each chapter provides a brief summary of the material, followed by a question and answer section. The chapter summaries highlight the major points and important information in each content category; the question and answer sections are fully explained and referenced, and cover all the information required by the ARRT for the mammography examination.

Chapters 6 and 7 each contain a complete practice mammography examination. The simulated examinations have been designed to reduce examination jitters by providing a true simulation of the actual certification examination. For the actual mammography examination, the ARRT allots 2½ hours to complete 115 questions. For each of these examinations, the examinee should plan to spend up to 2½ hours in a distraction-free environment to practice pacing and the economical use of time.

Olive Peart, MS, RT(R)(M)
Clinical Instructor
Program in Radiography
The Stamford Hospital
Stamford, Connecticut

Acknowledgments

In preparing this review book, I am indebted to Dorothy Saia, program director with the Radiography Program at Stamford Hospital in Stamford, Connecticut. Dorothy is the person most responsible for initiating the idea of a mammography review book and her suggestions, criticisms, corrections, and compliments provided invaluable help.

Special thanks go to those technologists who provided me with valuable insight and practical suggestions on the review questions. I wish to especially thank Pamela Hart, Katie Macari, and Carol Mackay.

Thanks also to my editors, Trish Casey, Catherine Johnson, and John Williams and to the copyeditors and other professionals at McGraw-Hill whose accuracy and suggestions helped me in the preparation of the final manuscript.

And finally, thanks to my husband and children whose reluctant understanding provided me the necessary freedom to compete this review manual. I know that they are as relieved as I am that this project is over.

As you (the student, mammographer, or technologist) use this text I hope you will e-mail me at peltrovijan@yahoo.com or contact me in writing at P.O. Box 13, Shrub Oak, NY 10588, with suggestions, changes, or additions, so that together we will strive to make mammography a fulfilling and rewarding profession for others.

Bibliography

This is a complete reference list of books and publications used in compiling the text and questions in this book. For your convenience, the last line of each answer refers back to the book or publication where the related information was found. For example, (Wentz, p. 7) refers to page 7 in the book *Mammography for Radiologic Technologists* by G. Wentz.

"Accreditation and Certification Overview." Feb. 2002. Food and Drug Administration (FDA) Internet. Accessed Feb. 2002. Available at **http://www.fda.gov/cdrh/mammography/robohelp/finalregs.htm**

American Cancer Society (ACS). *Breast Cancer Facts & Figures 1999–2000.* Atlanta, GA: American Cancer Society; 1999.

American College of Radiology (ACR). *Mammography Quality Control Manual.* Reston, VA: The American College of Radiology; 1999.

Andolina VF, Lille SL, Willison KM. *Mammographic Imaging: A Practical Guide.* Philadelphia: Lippincott Williams & Wilkins; 2001.

"Breast Cancer Resource Center: Benign Breast Conditions." 22 Sept. 1999. American Cancer Society. (ASC) Accessed Jan. 2000. Available at **http://cancer.org**

"Breast Cancer Resource Center: Detection & Symptoms." 22 Sept. 1999. American Cancer Society (ACS). Accessed Jan. 2000. Available at **http://cancer.org**

Bushong SC. *Radiologic Science for Technologists—Physics, Biology and Protection.* St. Louis, MO: Mosby; 2001.

Carlton RR, Adler AM. *Principles of Radiographic Imaging: An Art and a Science.* Albany, NY: Delmar; 2001.

Coon TA. MRI's role in assessing and managing breast disease. *Radiologic Technology* 67:311–336, 1996.

Harris JR, Lippman ME, Osborne CK. *Diseases of the Breast,* 2nd ed. Philadelphia: Lippincott Williams & Wilkins; 2000.

Lewis C. "Breast cancer: Better treatment saves more lives." *FDA Consumer* Jul.-Aug. 1999. U.S. Food and Drug Administration. Accessed Jan. 2001. Available at **http://www.fda.gov**

Logan-Young W, Hoffman NY. *Breast Cancer: A Practical Guide to Diagnosis.* Rochester, NY: Mt. Hope Publishing Co.; 1994.

Sanders R. *Clinical Sonography.* Philadelphia: Lippincott; 1998.

Tabár L, Dean PB. *Teaching Atlas of Mammography.* New York: Thieme; 1998.

Thomas CL. *Taber's Cyclopedic Medical Dictionary,* 18th ed. Philadelphia: F.A. Davis; 1997.

Tortora GJ, Grabowski SR. *Principles of Anatomy and Physiology.* New York: John Wiley & Sons; 2000.

Wentz G. *Mammography for Radiologic Technologists.* New York: McGraw-Hill; 1997.

CHAPTER 1

Patient Education and Assessment

Summary of Important Points

RISK FACTORS FOR BREAST CANCER

- The biggest risk factor for breast cancer is gender (female).

Other major factors include:

- *Aging:* A woman's risk of developing breast cancer increases with age.
- *Genetic risk factors:* About 10% of breast cancer cases are hereditary.
- *Family history of breast cancer:* Breast cancer risk is higher among women whose close blood relatives have this disease.
- *Personal history of breast cancer:* A woman with cancer in one breast has a greater risk of developing a new cancer in the other breast.

Minor risk factors that may slightly increase a woman's chance of developing breast cancer are:

- Not having children or having the first child at over age 30
- Not breast-feeding
- Early menarche (before age 12) or late menopause (after age 55)

BREAST DISEASE

Breast disease can be either benign or malignant.

Benign Breast Diseases

Like malignant conditions, benign diseases of the breast can manifest themselves physically, such as in a painful cyst or nipple discharge. Some breast diseases, however, can be detected only on the mammogram. Such breast disease will be seen as asymmetric densities, calcifications, circumscribed tumors, lesions, or skin thickening.

Malignant Diseases

The two main classifications of breast cancer are ductal and lobular carcinoma. Ductal carcinoma is the most common, occurring in about 90% of all cases. The classifications of ductal carcinoma are as follows:

- *Ductal carcinoma in situ:* the cancer is confined to the duct and does not invade the duct walls.
- *Invasive or infiltrating ductal carcinoma:* the cancer has spread from the ducts into the surrounding stromal tissue and may or may not extend into the pectoral fascia and muscle.

Lobular carcinoma affects 5–10% of all women.

- *Lobular carcinoma in situ* is not seen mammographically in 50% of cases; the abnormal cells grow within the lobules but do not penetrate through the lobule walls.
- *Invasive lobular carcinoma* is difficult to perceive on the radiographs; it may show as a spider web appearance or cause skin retraction.

Other Breast Carcinomas

Infiltrating medullary, colloid comedo, tubular, mucinous, papillary, and other carcinomas account for less than 10% of total breast cancer cases and have a better prognosis than infiltrating ductal or lobular cancers.

Appearance on Radiographs

Breast cancer may appear on the radiograph as asymmetric densities, calcifications, circumscribed tumors or lesions, or skin thickening.

- *Ductal calcifications* are granular- or casting-type calcifications and most often will appear in clusters.
- *Malignant circumscribed lesions* are ill-defined and high-density radiopaque, except for a

few rare carcinomas that are low-density radiopaque.

- *Skin thickening* will appear in cases of advanced breast cancer, small cancers in the axillary tail or behind the nipple, breast carcinoma in a large area, invasive comedocarcinoma, diffusely invasive ductal carcinoma (i.e., inflammatory carcinoma), secondary breast carcinoma, or metastasis from the opposite side.

DIAGNOSTIC OPTIONS

The mammogram remains the single most effective tool in the detection of breast cancer. There are, however, a number of adjunct diagnostic options:

- *Digital mammography* can be used with computer-aided diagnosis (CAD) to analyze digitized mammograms.
- *Three-dimensional color Doppler ultrasound* provides an anatomic display of blood flow.
- *Conventional ultrasound* is useful in determining whether the mass seen on the mammogram is solid versus cystic (malignant versus benign).
- *Magnetic resonance imaging* (MRI) technology is still developing. At present, the variety of imaging protocols chosen for breast imaging depends on the available hardware and software and will produce different results.
- *Breast scintigraphy* is a new technology, useful in detecting axillary node involvement. The sensitivity of the technique is limited with lesions under 1 cm.
- *Computed tomographic (CT) laser mammography* is an experimental technology that shows promise because no ionizing radiation is used. It can be used to differentiate cystic versus solid lesions and to image breast implants.
- *Nuclear medicine,* specifically using fluorodeoxyglucose (FDG) utilizes the need that cancer cells have for sugar. Because FDG is structurally similar to glucose, position-emitting isotopes will attach to FDG molecules. The technique called positron emission tomography (PET) scanning can be used to display an image of the tumor bed or to detect mediastinal lymph node metastases in breast cancer.
- *Miraluma* imaging of the breast is nuclear imaging using technetium Tc99m sestamibi.

Technetium Tc99m sestamibi, once injected into the blood stream, will concentrate in breast cancer cells. A gamma camera is used to examine where Technetium Tc99m sestamibi concentrated. Technetium Tc99m sestamibi is especially useful on patients with dense breasts, implants, diffuse calcifications, and breast tissue scarred by radiation or surgery.

- *Computerized thermal breast imaging* is a technology that has shown significant improvement in recent years. Thermal imaging may eventually reduce, if not replace, the need for surgical breast biopsy because of its effectiveness in predicting benign breast conditions. Because malignant lesions require a proliferation of blood vessels, thermal studies are able to outline areas of malignant growth as "hot" areas, versus the cooler areas of healthy breast tissue.
- *Sentinel node mapping* involves the injection of a radioactive tracer in the area around the tumor to identify the path to the lymph nodes that cancer cells take.

TREATMENT OPTIONS

Breast cancer can be treated with surgery, radiation, and drugs (chemotherapy and hormonal therapy). Doctors can use one or more of these treatments, depending on the type and location of the cancer, whether the disease has spread, and the patient's overall health status.

- *Lumpectomy* is the most breast-conserving surgery. It removes only the cancerous tissue and a surrounding margin of normal tissue.
- *Mastectomy* is the removal of the entire breast.
  - *A modified radical mastectomy* removes the entire breast and some of the underarm lymph nodes.
  - *A radical mastectomy* removes the entire breast, lymph nodes, and chest wall muscles under the breast. It is rarely performed today because the modified mastectomy is just as effective. The modified is also less debilitating and deforming.
- *Radiation therapy* is treatment with high-energy radiation to destroy cancer cells.
- *Chemotherapy* is an adjuvant therapy and involves the use of drugs to treat cancer that may have spread beyond the breast.
- Pain medication is available for patients in se-

vere pain from cancer. Newer pain medications are even more potent than morphine.

BREAST EXAMINATION

The American Cancer Society (ACS) guidelines for routine mammography screening are as follows:

- Women aged 40 and older should have a screening mammogram and a clinical breast examination (CBE) every year.
- Women between ages 20 and 39 should have a CBE every 3 years.
- Women aged 20 and older should perform a breast self-examination (BSE) every month.

Breast Self-Examination
A BSE should be performed monthly. It involves

- Looking for changes in the breast
- Feeling for changes in the breast

Clinical Breast Examination
A CBE is a check of the breast by a qualified health professional. A thorough clinical examination will locate any lumps or suspicious areas and any changes in the nipples or skin of the breast. The lymph nodes under the armpit and above the collarbone will also be checked for enlargement or firmness.

Medical History and Documentation
Medical and family history will provide information about symptoms and risk factors for breast cancer and benign breast conditions. The history should also include questions about other health problems.

Benefits and Risks of Mammography

Mortality Reduction
Breast cancer in its early stages is asymptomatic. Since the advent of modern mammography in the late 1960s, studies have conclusively proven that the mortality rate from breast cancer is significantly reduced with regular screening mammograms.

Risk From Radiation Exposure
A mammogram delivers very low doses of radiation. In general a screen-film mammogram will give about 0.1–0.2 rad average glandular dose when a grid is used.

Questions

1. The biggest risk factor for breast disease is

    (A) a family history of breast cancer
    (B) a personal history of breast cancer
    (C) gender
    (D) not breast-feeding

2. One of the minor risk factors for breast cancer could include

    (A) gender
    (B) aging
    (C) genetic risk factors
    (D) not breast-feeding

3. What is the approximate risk of developing breast cancer for a woman whose father's sister has the disease?

    (A) higher than normal risk
    (B) no significant change in risk
    (C) lower than normal risk
    (D) none of the above

4. Seventy-seven percent of breast cancers are discovered in women in which age group?

    (A) age 30 or under
    (B) over age 50
    (C) between ages 30 and 40
    (D) over age 20 but under age 30

5. Symptoms of benign breast disease not seen mammographically can include

    1. nipple discharge
    2. skin thickening
    3. circumscribed tumors

    (A) 1 only
    (B) 3 only
    (C) 2 and 3 only
    (D) 1 and 3 only

6. Symptoms of a malignant breast cancer can include

    1. skin thickening
    2. nipple discharge
    3. calcifications

    (A) 1 only
    (B) 2 and 3 only
    (C) 1 and 3 only
    (D) 1, 2, and 3

7. Skin thickening can be malignant but could also be caused by

    1. a breast abscess
    2. a calcified fibroadenoma
    3. postradiation

    (A) 1 only
    (B) 2 only
    (C) 1 and 2 only
    (D) 1 and 3 only

8. The two main classifications of breast cancer are

   1. ductal

   2. lobular

   3. medullary

     (A) 1 only

     (B) 2 only

     (C) 1 and 2 only

     (D) 1 and 3 only

9. Magnetic resonance imaging could be used

   1. as a primary breast cancer detection tool

   2. to image patients with breast implants to evaluate ruptures

   3. to determine tumor margins and the extent of tumor spread

     (A) 1 only

     (B) 1 and 2 only

     (C) 2 and 3 only

     (D) 1 and 3 only

10. Chemotherapy

     (A) involves the use of drugs to treat cancer that may have spread

     (B) is the destruction of cancer cells using high-energy radiation

     (C) involves mapping the area around a tumor with the injection of a radioactive tracer

     (D) is the removal of only the cancerous tissue from the breast

11. The American Cancer Society recommends that

   1. all women should have a screening mammogram every year

   2. women over 40 should have a screening mammogram every year

   3. new masses or lumps in the breast should be checked by a health care provider

     (A) 1 only

     (B) 2 only

     (C) 1 and 3 only

     (D) 2 and 3 only

12. A health care provider should evaluate which of the following breast changes?

   1. lumps or swellings

   2. skin irritation or dimpling

   3. milky discharge from the nipple

     (A) 1 only

     (B) 1 and 2 only

     (C) 2 and 3 only

     (D) 1, 2, and 3

13. A clinical breast examination (CBE) should be performed every

   1. year after age 40

   2. 3 years between ages 20 and 39

   3. month after age 50

     (A) 1 only

     (B) 2 only

     (C) 1 and 2 only

     (D) 2 and 3 only

14. A CBE can be performed by which of the following?

   1. the radiologist

   2. the patient

   3. a healthcare professional

     (A) 1 only

     (B) 2 only

     (C) 2 and 3 only

     (D) 1 and 3 only

15. A breast self-examination (BSE) should be done regularly by

   1. the radiologist

   2. the patient

   3. a healthcare professional

     (A) 1 only

     (B) 2 only

     (C) 2 and 3 only

     (D) 1 and 3 only

16. All women over the age of _____ should perform a BSE regularly.

    (A) 20
    (B) 30
    (C) 40
    (D) 50

17. The two-step method of BSE is to

    (A) look and feel for changes in the breast
    (B) examine your breasts and have a regular mammogram
    (C) check for lumps in the breast and keep a journal of changes in the breast
    (D) examine your breasts and nipples

18. When visually inspecting the breast, the changes that should be recorded include

    1. changes in size and shape
    2. changes in texture or color
    3. indentations

       (A) 1 and 2 only
       (B) 2 and 3 only
       (C) 1 and 3 only
       (D) 1, 2, and 3

19. The patient's medical history and documentation will

    1. provide the radiologist with information about risk factors for breast cancer
    2. give the radiologist information about symptoms of breast cancer
    3. provide information about possible benign breast conditions

       (A) 1 and 2 only
       (B) 2 and 3 only
       (C) 1 and 3 only
       (D) 1, 2, and 3

20. The importance of BSE and a CBE is stressed because

    1. both will detect benign breast diseases, which are very common
    2. both will help in the detection of malignant breast conditions
    3. a mammogram is not 100% effective

       (A) 1 only
       (B) 2 only
       (C) 2 and 3 only
       (D) 1 and 3 only

21. Which of the following are methods used in BSEs?

    1. using the pads of the three middle fingers to palpate the entire breast
    2. palpating around the breast in circular patterns
    3. using up and down lines or wedge patterns during palpation

       (A) 1 only
       (B) 1 and 2 only
       (C) 1 and 3 only
       (D) 1, 2, and 3

22. For a menstruating woman, when is the best time of the month to perform a BSE?

    (A) one week before the start of menstruation
    (B) on the 1st day of the month
    (C) on the last day of the month
    (D) one week after the end of menstruation

23. A BSE can be done

    1. while standing
    2. in the shower
    3. lying down

       (A) 1 only
       (B) 2 only
       (C) 2 and 3 only
       (D) 1, 2, and 3

24. During a BSE, standing upright makes it easier to examine the

    (A) upper and outer parts of the breast
    (B) inner and lower parts of the breast
    (C) nipple area of the breast
    (D) subareola area of the breast

25. The first step in evaluating a woman with suspected breast cancer is a

    (A) lesson on BSE and a breast ultrasound
    (B) mammogram and a lesson on breast self examination
    (C) CBE and a mammogram
    (D) complete medical history and CBE

26. During a CBE, lumps or masses in the armpit may indicate the spread of breast cancer to

    1. lymph nodes in the axilla
    2. lymph nodes above the collarbone
    3. lymph nodes in the arm

       (A) 1 only
       (B) 3 only
       (C) 1 and 2
       (D) 2 and 3

27. In mammography the radiation dose per view is generally about

    (A) 0.1–0.2 rad
    (B) 1.0–2.0 rad
    (C) 0.01–0.02 rad
    (D) 2–3 mrad

28. In which age group is the radiosensitivity of the breast the greatest?

    (A) between 20 and 35
    (B) between 40 and 50
    (C) between 55 and 60
    (D) over 70

29. The 5-year survival rate for a patient with a stage 0 breast cancer is about

    (A) 49%
    (B) 76%
    (C) 88%
    (D) 100%

30. During a mammogram, which of the following will affect the average glandular dose per breast?

    1. degree of breast compression
    2. the HVL of the x-ray beam
    3. breast size and composition

       (A) 1 only
       (B) 2 only
       (C) 3 only
       (D) 1, 2, and 3

Answers and Explanations

1. **(C)** Risk factors increase a woman's risk for breast cancer. Risk factors are divided into major and minor. Major risks are those outside of a woman's control, such as gender and age. Minor risks are those within a woman's control, such as use of oral contraceptives. Simply being a woman is the main risk factor for developing breast cancer. Breast cancer can affect men, but this disease is much more common among women than men. *(Breast Cancer Resource Center: Prevention and Risk Facors, pp. 1–8; Wentz, pp. 7–8)*

2. **(D)** A risk factor is anything that increases a person's chance of getting a disease. Major risk factors cannot be changed. Minor factors are linked to cancer-causing factors in the environment or may be related to personal choices, such as breast-feeding. *(Breast Cancer Resource Center: Prevention and Risk Factors, pp. 1–8; Wentz, p. 8)*

3. **(A)** Major risk factors carry a significantly higher risk for breast cancer than minor risk factors. Breast cancer risk would therefore be higher among women whose close blood relatives have the disease. Blood relatives can be either from the mother's or father's side of the family. *(Breast Cancer Resource Center: Prevention and Risk Factors, pp. 1–8)*

4. **(B)** A woman's risk of developing breast cancer increases with age. Older women have the greatest risk. Women younger than age 30 years account for only 0.3% of breast cancer cases, and women in their 30s account for about 3.5% of cases. *(Breast Cancer Resource Center: Prevention and Risk Factors, pp. 1–8; Wentz, p. 8)*

5. **(A)** Whereas skin thickening or tumors will be seen on a mammogram, nipple discharge is not seen mammographically. Most nipple discharges or secretions are not cancerous. In general, if the secretion appears clear or milky, yellow or green, cancer is very unlikely. Further testing such as a ductogram or galactogram helps in determining the cause of nipple discharge. *(Breast Cancer Resource Center: Benign Breast Conditions, pp. 1–6; Tabár, pp. 16–20)*

6. **(D)** Unfortunately, breast cancer in its early states is symptomless. As the cancer grows, some symptoms may appear. These symptoms can include lumps in the breast, thickening of the breast skin, puckering or dimpling of the breast, inverted nipples, or a discharge from the nipples. *(Andolina, pp. 139–161)*

7. **(D)** Skin thickening or lymphedema of the breast usually indicates cancer, but may also be because of a breast abscess located behind the nipple, mediastinal blockage due to sarcoidosis (advanced stages), Hodgkin disease, lung cancer, bronchial cancer with mediastinal metastases, esophageal cancer with mediastinal metastases, right heart failure, advanced gynecologic malignancy, or postoperative or postradiation lymphedema. *(Tabár, p. 241)*

8. **(C)** Ductal carcinoma occurs in 90% of all women with breast cancer. Lobular carcinoma affects 5–10% of women with breast cancer. Other forms of breast carcinoma, such as medullary, account for less than 10% of the total breast cancer cases. *(Breast Cancer Resources: Detection and Symptoms, pp. 7–11)*

9. **(C)** At present, MRI technology is still developing. The results produced from MRI imaging will depend on the available hardware and software and the variety of imaging protocols. Because of the cost of the MRI and the developing nature of the technology, MRI cannot be used as a screening tool. MRI, however, is useful for evaluating ruptures, leaks, free silicone in the surrounding breast tissue, or the formation of silicone granulomas. Also, the tumor margins and the extent of tumor spread are often better defined on the MRI than on mammography. *(Coon, pp. 311–336; Wentz pp. 9–10)*

10. **(A)** Chemotherapy involves the use of drugs to treat cancer that may have spread beyond the breast. The chemotherapy treatments may last 3–6 months depending on the intensity of the chemotherapy drug and how far the cancer has spread. Generally, chemotherapy treatment is given in cycles, with a period of treatment followed by a recovery period. *(ACS, p. 3; Lewis, pp. 1–4)*

11. **(D)** The guidelines as suggested by the ACS are:
    * Women aged 40 and older should have a screening mammogram and CBE every year.
    * Women between ages 20 and 39 should have a CBE every 3 years.
    * Women aged 20 and older should perform a BSE every month.
    * All lumps or suspicious areas and any changes in the nipple or skin of the breast should be reported to a healthcare provider. *(ACS, p. 11; Breast Cancer Resource Center: Detection and Symptoms, p. 1)*

12. **(B)** Changes such as a lump or swelling, tenderness, skin irritation or dimpling, or nipple pain or retraction should be evaluated as soon as possible. In general, if the nipple discharge is clear or milky, yellow, or green a cancer is unlikely. If the discharge is red or red-brown, suggesting blood, it could be due to either a malignant or a benign condition. *(Breast Cancer Resource: Detection and Symptoms pp. 1–5)*

13. **(C)** A CBE is an examination of the breast by a healthcare professional such as a physician, nurse-practitioner, nurse, or physician assistant. Between ages 20 and 39, women should have a CBE every 3 years. After age 40, women should have a CBE every year. *(ACS, p. 11; Breast Cancer Resource: Detection and Symptoms, pp. 1–3)*

14. **(D)** A CBE is an examination of the breast by a healthcare professional such as a radiologist, physician, nurse-practitioner, nurse, or physician assistant. The same examination, performed by the patient on herself, is referred to as the BSE. *(ACS, p. 11; Breast Cancer Resource: Detection and Symptoms, pp. 1–3)*

15. **(B)** A BSE should be done by the patient, 1 week after the menstrual period ends, when the breasts are not tender or swollen. For women not having regular menstruation, the BSE should be done on the same day every month. *(ACS, p. 11; Breast Cancer Resource: Detection and Symptoms, p. 3)*

16. **(A)** Because a small percentage of cancers can be missed by mammography, all women over age 20 should perform a BSE every month. These guidelines are for women with no symptoms of breast cancer and who have not been identified to be at a higher risk for breast cancer. *(ACS, p. 11; Breast Cancer Resource: Detection and Symptoms, p. 1)*

17. **(A)** For BSE, the first step is to look for changes, either while standing or sitting. A check should be made for indentations, retracted nipples, dimpling, or prolonged skin conditions. The next step is to feel for changes using light, medium, and firm pressure and the pads of three fingers in either in a circular, up-and-down line, or wedge pattern. The entire breast must be checked (Figure 1–1). *(ACS, p. 13; Breast Cancer Resource Center: Detection and Symptoms, pp. 2–3)*

18. **(D)** The visual stage of a BSE is a check for signs of breast cancer. These signs can include changes in size, texture, or color of the breast; prolonged skin irritation; redness or

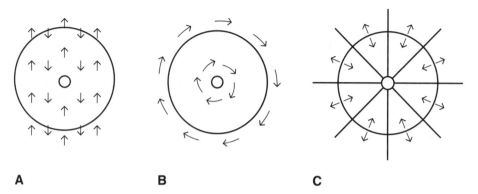

A   **B**   **C**

Figure 1–1. Breast self-examination (BSE) patterns showing (A) vertical, (B) circular, and (C) wedge patterns of BSE.

scaliness; dimpling; or nipple retraction. *(Breast Cancer Resource: Detection and Symptoms, pp. 1–3)*

19. (D) The medical history will provide information about the patient's symptoms and any other health problems and risk factors for benign or malignant breast conditions. *(Breast Cancer Resource: Detection and Symptoms, p. 4)*

20. (C) Although the BSE and the CBE can detect benign breast conditions, they are primarily important as complimentary tests. Both the BSE and CBE will compliment the mammogram and help in the detection of breast cancers. Unfortunately, the mammogram is not foolproof. Even under ideal conditions the mammogram will not find all breast cancers 100% of the time. *(ACS, p. 11; Breast Cancer: Detection and Symptoms, p. 4; Wentz, p. 7)*

21. (D) Feeling for changes in the breast involves using light, medium, and firm pressure. The pads of three fingers are used in either a circular, up-and-down line, or wedge pattern. The entire breast must be checked. *(ACS, p. 13; Breast Cancer Resource Center: Detection and Symptoms, pp. 2–3)*

22. (D) The patient should perform a BSE 1 week after the menstrual period ends, when

the breasts are not tender or swollen. *(ACS, p. 11; Breast Cancer Resource: Detection and Symptoms, p. 3)*

23. (D) A BSE should be done either sitting or standing in front of a mirror; standing upright makes it easier to examine the upper and outer parts of the breast, but the breast must also be examined while lying down. Because the fingers glide more easily over wet skin, the breast can be checked while in the shower. Large-breasted women should examine their breasts while lying on their side. *(Breast Cancer Resource: Detection and Symptoms, pp. 1–4)*

24. (A) A BSE should be done either sitting or standing in front of a mirror; standing upright makes it easier to examine the upper and outer parts of the breast, but the breast must also be examined while lying down. *(Breast Cancer Resource: Detection and Symptoms, pp. 1–4)*

25. (D) The first step in evaluating a woman with suspected breast cancer is a complete medical history and physical or clinical examination. The medical history will provide information about the patient's symptoms and any other health problems and risk factors for benign or malignant breast conditions. A clinical examination will be done to locate any lump or suspicious areas and to examine the texture, size, and shape of the breast. Once the medical and clinical examinations are completed, biopsies or imaging tests such as mammography can be performed if indicated. *(Breast Cancer Resource: Detection and Symptoms, p. 4)*

26. **(C)** In a CBE special attention should be given to any lumps, whether they are attached to the skin or deeper tissue. Breast cancer will leave the breast via the lymph nodes; therefore, any obvious enlargement of nodes in the axilla (under the arm) or above the collarbone must be evaluated. *(Breast Cancer Resource: Detection and Symptoms, pp. 1–4)*

27. **(A)** The ACR recommends that the average glandular dose on the mammogram be no greater than 0.3 rads (300 mrad or 3 mGy) with a grid or 0.1 rad (100 mrad or 1 mGy) without a grid. With modern mammography equipment the patient will usually receive only about 0.1–0.2 rads per view. *(Andolina, p. 34; Bushong, p. 553)*

28. **(A)** The breasts of young women are generally denser than those of older women. Younger breasts will therefore require more radiation to penetrate and will absorb more radiation than those of older women. Fortunately, the incidence of breast cancer in this age group is very low. *(Andolina, p. 25; Wentz, p. 8)*

29. **(D)** A pathologist looks at the tissue sample under a microscope and assigns a grade to it. The grade helps to predict the patient's prognosis—the lower the grade the slower growing the cancer. Five-year survival rate refers to the percent of patients who live at least 5 years after their cancer is diagnosed. Many of these patients live much longer than 5 years after diagnosis, but 5-year rates are used to produce a standard way of discussing prognosis. Five-year rates will exclude from the calculations patients dying of other diseases and is considered to be a more accurate way to describe the prognosis for patients with a particular type and stage of cancer (Table 1–1). *(Breast Cancer Resource: Detection and Symptoms, p. 11; Lewis, pp. 5–6)*

TABLE 1–1. BREAST CANCER SURVIVAL BY STAGE

Stage		5-Year Relative Survival Rate
0	Carcinoma in situ	100%
I	Tumor ≤2 cm; axillary node negative	98%
IIA, IIB	Tumor 2–5 cm with or without positive nodes or >5 cm without positive nodes	88%, 76%
IIIA, IIIB	>5 cm with positive nodes	
	Any size if spread to breast skin, chest wall, or internal breast lymph nodes	56%, 49%
IV	Any size if there is distant metastasis (e.g., to bone, lungs)	16%

30. **(D)** The major factors affecting dose are:
    - *The imaging chain*—the screen/film combination, and processing environment.
    - *The x-ray beam energy*—the higher the kVp and half-value layer (HVL) the lower the patient dose
    - *The compression*—greater compression will result in decreased exposure and therefore decreased dose
    - The patient's breast tissue type (composition) and thickness—denser glandular breast requires more exposure than fatter breast *(Wentz, pp. 119–120)*

CHAPTER 2

Instrumentation and Quality Assurance

Summary of Important Points

DESIGN CHARACTERISTICS OF FILM-SCREEN MAMMOGRAPHY UNITS

All mammography units are designed to image the soft tissue of the breast while displaying the necessary subtle contrast differences. Older mammography generators were three-phase generators; all modern generators are high-frequency generators. Like the older units, these rectify the input to produce a direct current (DC) voltage waveform, but the modern high-frequency generators essentially provide a constant potential with about 1% ripple. The high frequency allows more efficient x-ray production and therefore produces a higher effective energy x-ray beam. The result is higher x-ray output for a given kVp and mA setting.

kVp range

The kVp range will depend on the target/filtration material available.

- Molybdenum (Mo) target tube: 24–30 kVp
- Rhodium (Rh) target tube: 26–32 kVp
- Tungsten (W) target tube: 22–26 kVp

The kVp use will depend on a number of factors (e.g., radiologist preference, equipment calibration, manufacturer's recommendations, equipment design, characteristic curve of the screen-film combination, processing, and patient breast size and thickness). The kVp will have a major effect on exposure time and dose.

The kVp selection can affect the radiographic contrast because contrast is highest in thinner breasts and lowest in thicker breasts. In the thicker breast more radiation is needed (more kVp) and there is greater tissue absorption of the low-kVp radiation. Increased kVp will lower dose but reduce contrast. Decreased kVp will increase dose and increase contrast.

MAMMOGRAPHY TUBE (ANODE, FILTRATION, WINDOW)

In mammography, special target materials and filtrations are combined to provide the low-energy beam needed. The target-filter combination will essentially shape the x-ray beam providing the necessary kVp range to penetrate dense or fatty breast. Common combinations include

- Molybdenum target with 0.03 mm molybdenum filtration
- Rhodium target with 0.025 mm rhodium filtration
- Molybdenum and tungsten target with molybdenum and rhodium filtration
- Molybdenum and rhodium target with molybdenum and rhodium filtration

The material used for the exit port or window of the x-ray tube is borosilicate glass or beryllium (Be). A regular glass window would harden the emerging beam by eliminating the soft characteristic radiation.

The intensity of the beam is less on the anode side than on the cathode side because of the anode heel effect. The cathode-side output of the x-ray tube is always directed to the base; that is, the thickness area of the breast.

COMPRESSION DEVICES

Compression in mammography is provided by a flat-surfaced compression paddle. Important design characteristics are:

- the flat surface must be parallel to film receptor.
- the chest wall edge of the compression paddle should not extend beyond the chest wall edge of the image receptor by more than 1% of the SID.
- a shadow of the vertical edge of the compression paddle should not be visible on the image.
- the lip along the chest wall should be 2–4 cm in height.
- the lip should have a right angle at the chest wall.

AUTOMATIC EXPOSURE CONTROL

Automatic exposure control (AEC) is used in modern mammography units. AEC controls the length of the exposure and will therefore determine the density of the final image. Two types of AEC devices are found in modern mammography units:

- the ionization chamber
- the solid-state diode

Underexposure is still a common problem in mammography and occurs when the AEC cell is not placed over the densest area of the breast.

GRIDS

Grids are used to improve radiographic contrast by decreasing the amount of scattered radiation that reaches the image receptor. Mammography grids are thinner than conventional grids. The interspace material may be carbon fiber, wood, or other low-attenuation interspacing instead of the aluminum that is used in general radiography grids. All modern mammographic units have moving grids, but they only move in one direction and do not reciprocate. The grid ratios can vary from 3:1 to 5:1, focused to the SID for increased contrast. Grid frequencies of 30–50 lines per centimeter are common. The use of grids will always result in increased dose to the patient. There is a new high transmission cellular (HTC) grid with characteristics of a crossed grid. It can reduce scatter in two directions rather than the one direction of the linear or focused grid. These grids use copper not lead as the grid strip, and air rather than wood or aluminum for the interspace material. The physical

dimensions result in a grid ratio of 3.8:1 and when compared to a similar ratio linear grid the HTC grids result in equal or less radiation dose to the patient.

BEAM RESTRICTION DEVICES

Beam-restricting or -limiting devices are cones, collimators, or diaphragms used to regulate the size and shape of the x-ray beam. There are three facts to consider when using beam-restricting devices.

- The entire film should be exposed (extraneous light will compromise the perception of fine detail).
- Collimation should not extend beyond any edge of the image receptor by more than 2% of the SID.
- Decreasing the x-ray field will require an increase in exposure to maintain constant density.

SYSTEM GEOMETRY (SID, OID, MAGNIFICATION)

Focal Spot Size
The recommended focal spot sizes in mammography are:

- 0.4 mm or smaller for routine work (the most commonly used is 0.3 mm).
- 0.15 mm or smaller for magnification (the most common focal spot size in magnification is 0.1 mm).

Size and shape of the focal spot are determined by the

- size and shape of electron beam hitting the anode.
- design and relationship of the filament coil to the focusing cup.
- angle of the anode.

SID
In mammography the aim is to have the smallest focal spot coupled with the longest SID. The recommended SID in mammography is 50–80 cm.

OID
The object to image-receptor distance should be as small as possible. The only exception is microfocus magnification views. Magnification will reduce

scatter, but the greater the magnification factor the greater the skin dose to the patient. Also, magnification decreases resolution. A common magnification factor is 1.5 times. Other factors can be 1.6, 1.7, 1.85, or 2 times. Factors affecting resolution and sharpness are

- motion due to long exposure times.
- poor screen-film contact.
- increase in the focal spot size.
- increase in the object-to-image receptor distance (OID).
- decrease in the source-to-image receptor distance (SID).
- the relationship between the OID and the SID.
- characteristics of the screen (faster screens exhibit greater unsharpness).

IMAGING COMPONENTS

The screen-film system is the most commonly used imaging recording system in mammography today. However, digital mammography is now available and its use will undoubtedly spread in the coming years.

Film
The film is used to record the image, display the image, and provide archival storage. Mammography films are single emulsion and high contrast. High-contrast films generally have limited exposure latitude resulting in poor contrast, but many current mammography films now have significantly higher inherent contrast. Other film characteristics such as speed must also be taken into account to reduce patient dose.

Screens
Single-screen cassette systems are used in mammography to provide the best resolution.

Cassettes or Image Recorders
The cassette or film holder holds and stores the film during exposure. The newer, thinner cassettes are designed for both daylight and regular systems and have an identification system slot, capable of recording patient information on the film.

DIGITAL MAMMOGRAPHY

Full-field digital mammography (FFDM) uses an amorphous silicon-based flat panel detector. X-rays will react with the detector or imaging plate (IP) to form a latent image. The electronic system of the digital unit will collect a digital readout of the latent image. This image information can be electronically transmitted, manipulated, and efficiently stored using a variety of methods. With digital imaging, the cassette has been replaced by the detector and electronic system. Some of these cassette-less systems utilize a 1-mm thick sheet of glass coated with cesium iodide plus an amorphous silicone detector. The cesium iodide is used to absorb x-rays and the silicon chips will detect the x-ray photons. Digital mammography can also be combined with the new computer-assisted diagnosis (CAD) technology. Here, a computer can in effect preread the mammograms, identifying areas of suspicion or areas needing additional workup. Digital imaging can also be combined with a picture achieving and communication system (PACS) enabling teleradiography and filmless libraries, which can be accessed via telephone, the Internet, or any other off-site location.

QUALITY ASSURANCE

Quality assurance and processor quality control are absolutely essential in producing quality images. Guidelines determined by the Mammography Quality Standards Act and the American College of Radiology provide the standard criteria. These criteria exceed the criteria for processing of radiographic studies done in a diagnostic radiology department.

MAMMOGRAPHER TEST	FREQUENCY
Darkroom cleanliness	Daily
Processor quality control	Daily
Mobile unit quality control	Daily
Screen cleanliness	Weekly
View boxes and viewing conditions	Weekly
Phantom images	Weekly
Visual checklist	Monthly
Repeat/reject analysis	Quarterly
Analysis of fixer retention in film	Quarterly

Darkroom fog	Semiannually
Screen-film contact	Semiannually
Compression	Semiannually

MEDICAL PHYSICIST TEST   ALL TESTS ARE
                                DONE ANNUALLY

Mammographic unit assembly
  evaluation
Collimation assessment (field
  light and x-ray congruence)
Evaluation of system resolution
AEC system performance
Uniformity of screen speed
Artifact evaluation
Image quality evaluation
kVp accuracy and
  reproducibility
Beam quality assessment
Breast exposure and AEC
  reproducibility
Average glandular dose
Radiation output rate
Measure of view-box luminance
  and room illuminance

TESTING DETAILS

Darkroom Cleanliness

The purpose of darkroom cleanliness is to minimize artifacts on radiographs due to bits of dust,
dirt, or food between the screen and film. This is
extremely important when using single emulsion
film, as in mammography, not only because they
are more obvious, but because they can look like
microcalcifications and lead to misdiagnosis or repeat examinations.

Processor Quality Control

Processor quality control should be carried out
daily, at the beginning of the day before processing
any films. This test will confirm and verify that the
processor-chemical system is working properly according to specifications.

  Required: A 21-step sensitometer and a densitometer.

  Processor quality control records should be
saved for 1 year. Sensitometric films should be
saved for the last full month.

Screen Cleanliness

Screens should be cleaned at least weekly, but also
anytime dust or other artifacts are noted by the
mammographer or radiologist.

Illuminators/Viewing Conditions

Viewing conditions can be extremely critical in
mammography. High luminance view boxes with
proper masking of each film are essential. Typically,
view boxes should have a luminance level of approximately 1500 candela per square meter (cd/m²).
For mammography, the luminance level should be
at least 3500 cd/m². (The unit candela per meter is
sometimes referred to as the "nit.")

Phantom Images

Phantom images are taken to ensure that film density, contrast, uniformity, and image quality are
maintained at optimum levels.

  Required: A mammographic phantom (4- to 4.5-
cm thick tissue equivalent breast phantom), with
an acrylic disc 4 mm thick permanently fixed on
the phantom, in a position that does not obscure
any phantom detail.

  Note: The mammographic phantom should always be viewed by the same person, on the same
view box, under the same viewing conditions, using the same type of magnifying glass at the same
time of day.

Visual Checklist

This test is performed to ensure the mechanical in-
tegrity and safety of the mammographic equipment and accessory devices. The system indicator
lights, displays, mechanical locks, and detents are
all checked.

Reject/Repeat Analysis

The overall repeat rate ideally should not exceed
2%, but a rate lower than 5% is acceptable once the
quality assurance program is operational. To be sta-
tistically meaningful, a volume of at least 250 patients needs to be measured. The percentage of repeats from each category should be close. If one
category is significantly higher than the others, it
should be targeted for improvement.

Analysis of Fixer Retention in Film

The amount of fixer (hypo) retention in any processed film is an indication of the length of time

that film will retain its archival quality (image quality). Excess residual fixer can degrade the quality of the image.

Required: Residual hypo test solution, available commercially, or hypo estimator (e.g., Kodak Hypo Estimator, publication N-405, or equivalent).

If there is an excess of hypo retained on the film, the processor wash tanks and water flow rates, in addition to fixer replenishment rates, need to be assessed.

Darkroom Fog

This test is performed to ensure that the film is not fogged as a result of cracks in the safelight or other light sources in and out of the darkroom.

Required: Mammographic or routine x-ray unit, densitometer, a radiopaque card, and a watch or timer.

Screen/Film Contact and Identification

It is important to be able to identify each screen-cassette combination. If a problem occurs with one of the cassettes, for example, if an artifact is detected in one of the cassettes, appropriate identification will allow the mammographer to locate the cassette and correct the problem. Each screen should be marked with a unique identification number near the left or right edge of the screen, using a marker approved by the screen manufacturer. The same identification number should be placed on the outside of each cassette.

Required: Mammographic film, a densitometer, and copper wire mesh screens with at least 40 wires per inch grid density. These are commercially available. The mesh can be placed between two thin sheets of acrylic to protect it.

The optical density of the final image must be measured using a densitometer with at least a 2-mm diameter aperture. The density should be between 0.70 and 0.80 when measured near the chest wall side of the film. A thin sheet of acrylic can be placed near the x-ray tube window to adjust the density to the ideal level.

Any cassette having a large area (greater than 1 cm in diameter) of poor contact that cannot be eliminated should be replaced. Multiple small areas of poor contact are considered acceptable.

Compression

This test ensures that the mammographic system can provide adequate compression in both manual and automatic mode, and that too much compression cannot be applied. The compression should be adequate to separate glandular tissue without causing injury to the patient or damage to the compression device.

Required: Bathroom scale and several towels.

Adequate compression ranges from 25–40 lb in automatic mode (111–200 Newtons). The initial automatic compression should not exceed 45 lb of pressure.

MAMMOGRAPHY QUALITY STANDARDS ACT

Accreditation and Certification

The Mammography Quality Standards Act (MQSA) was enacted on October 27, 1992, to establish minimal national quality standards for mammography.

Agencies: The Food and Drug Administration (FDA) and the "States as Certifiers" (SAC) are the only organizations authorized to issue MQSA certification.

Process: Before a mammography facility can legally perform mammograms, it must be certified. The facility must first contact an accreditation body. Provisional certification (valued for 6 months) is usually issued by the FDA as soon as the accreditation has been accepted. The accreditation body will then collect clinical images and other data to complete the accreditation process.

Regulations

All technologists performing mammograms must meet the training requirements of the MQSA. Each mammogram facility must have a written policy for collecting and resolving consumer complaints. If the facility is unable to resolve a complaint, the consumer must be given instructions on how to file complaints with the facility's accreditation body.

Record Keeping: Mammography films and medical records of patients must be kept for a period of not less than 5 years, or not less than 10 years if no additional mammograms of the patient are performed at the facility (longer if mandated by state or local law).

Communication of Results: All facilities must send each patient a summary of the mammography report written in lay terms within 30 days of the mammographic examination.

Medical Audit: All facilities must keep a medical outcomes audit to follow positive mammography results and to correlate pathology results with the interpreting physician's findings.

Questions

1. In mammography, selecting extremely low kVp values

    (A) reduces contrast and lowers patient dose
    (B) increases contrast but increases patient dose
    (C) reduces contrast but increases patient dose
    (D) increases contrast and reduces patient dose

2. What target filtration-combination provides the best penetration for dense or thick breast?

    (A) molybdenum target with molybdenum filtration
    (B) rhodium target with rhodium filtration
    (C) tungsten target with tungsten filtration
    (D) molybdenum target with appropriate K-edge filtration

3. The material used for the exit port of the mammography tube is necessary because

    (A) the intensity of the beam is less on the anode side than on the cathode side
    (B) regular glass would harden the emerging beam
    (C) the intensity of the beam is more on the anode side than the cathode side
    (D) regular glass would soften the emerging beam

4. The intensity of the x-ray beam from the cathode side of the tube is generally higher because

    (A) soft characteristic radiation emerges from the anode side
    (B) the cathode side is directed to the thickest part of the breast
    (C) the heel effect causes variation in the intensity of the x-ray beam
    (D) the heel effect hardens the beam at the anode side

5. The design of the lip of the compression paddle (both height and angle along the chest wall) affects all of the following EXCEPT that it

    (A) prevents the posterior and axillary fat from overlapping the body of the breast
    (B) allows uniform compression of the posterior breast tissue
    (C) helps to increase structural strength of the compression paddle
    (D) ensures even compression of the anterior breast tissue

6. The *primary* goal of compression is to

    (A) reduce the object-to-image receptor distance of the lesion
    (B) allow uniform penetration of structures within the breast
    (C) reduce the possibility of motion during the exposure
    (D) reduce the radiation dose to the breast

7. AEC failure, resulting in an underexposed film, can be caused by

(A) processing deficiencies such as fluctuating developer temperature
(B) improper placement of the dense breast tissue/size over the detector
(C) decreased radiographic contrast
(D) inadequate breast compression

8. Most AEC circuitry in modern mammographic imaging has at least three detectors. Three or more detectors are recommended because

(A) multiple detectors allow for maximum variations in breast size and tissue density
(B) AEC detectors eliminate the guesswork in determining the proper exposure factor for each patient
(C) detectors have the ability to terminate the exposure by back-up timer when a maximum exposure time or maximum mAs is reached
(D) all AEC detector systems provide consistent film densities because of the high-contrast mammography films

9. The major difference between the general radiography grid and the grid used in mammography is that the

(A) grid use in general radiography causes an increase in exposure
(B) grids in general radiography have higher ratios
(C) use of a grid in mammography increases patient dose
(D) grids in mammography improve the radiographic image contrast

10. The grid ratio can vary in modern mammography units. A common grid ratio used is

(A) 7:1
(B) 6:1
(C) 5:1
(D) 4:1

11. As the size of the x-ray field decreases, to maintain a constant image density the exposure will

(A) increase
(B) decrease
(C) not change significantly
(D) decrease inversely

12. The chest wall edge of the compression paddle should be aligned just beyond the chest wall edge of the image receptor to

(A) avoid pushing the patient's chest away and losing breast tissue
(B) properly position and compress the breast
(C) permit uniform exposure and reduce patient discomfort
(D) avoid projecting the chest wall edge of the paddle on the mammogram

13. Which of the following affects focal spot size?

(A) angle of the anode
(B) a decrease in the source-to-image receptor distance
(C) decreasing the size of the collimated beam
(D) changing the relationship between the OID and the SID

14. In mammography the commonly used focal spot size for routine work is

(A) 0.4 mm
(B) 0.3 mm
(C) 0.2 mm
(D) 0.1 mm

15. Which of the following characteristics are unique to mammography cassettes?

(A) must be easy to open
(B) should be durable
(C) generally have a single intensifying screen
(D) should have low absorption characteristics

16. Two main disadvantages of extended processing are

    (A) decreased film speed and increased film fog
    (B) increased film speed and decreased film fog
    (C) increased processing artifact and increased film fog
    (D) decreased processing artifact and increased film speed

17. In digital mammography both the film and cassette can be replaced by

    (A) a detector and electronic system
    (B) the CAD technology system
    (C) a flexible storage phosphor
    (D) photostimulatable plates

18. The greatest difference between digital technology and conventional mammography imaging is

    (A) the higher resolution increases the patient dose in digital technology
    (B) there is no latent image formation when using digital technology
    (C) in digital technology, the final image can be manipulated
    (D) the image can never be displayed on a film in digital technology

19. All of the following are characteristics of double emulsion film/screens combination. Which characteristic makes these systems undesirable in mammography use?

    (A) They are less susceptible to imaging dust and dirt than the single emulsion systems.
    (B) They do not require extended processing times to develop optimum contrast and speed.
    (C) The screens are very efficient at converting x-ray energy to visible or ultraviolet light.
    (D) The system has a lower resolution than the single emulsion systems.

20. Film fog is best demonstrated on the characteristic curve as

    (A) the straight-line portion of the graph
    (B) the toe of the graph
    (C) the shoulder of the graph
    (D) the shift of the graph to the left

21. The characteristic curve, obtained by plotting density values from a sensitometer, can be used to assess all of the following EXCEPT

    (A) to compare two different types of films
    (B) to compare the same film under different processing conditions
    (C) to compare the x-ray beam quality with different films
    (D) to monitor the daily processing conditions

22. The characteristic curve of two films is plotted. The curve of film (A) is positioned to the left of the curve of film (B).

    1. film A is faster than film B
    2. film B is faster than film A
    3. at any optical density, film A will require less exposure than film B

    (A) 1 only
    (B) 2 only
    (C) 2 and 3 only
    (D) 1 and 3 only

23. Which of the following mammographic quality control tests is performed monthly?

    (A) phantom images
    (B) visual checklist
    (C) repeat analysis
    (D) screen cleanliness

24. Adequate "air bleed time" refers to the

    (A) elapsed time between film loading and exposure
    (B) time taken to release air from the processor drain tank
    (C) time taken to remove air from the water tank
    (D) resolution time of screens

25. Which of the following quality control tests does NOT require a densitometer?

    (A) darkroom fog
    (B) screen-film contact
    (C) screen cleanliness
    (D) phantom images

26. The criteria to pass the ACR Mammography Accreditation on phantom imaging requires a minimum of _____ masses.

    (A) two
    (B) three
    (C) four
    (D) five

27. In establishing processing quality control operating levels, the medium density is designated as the density

    (A) closest to but not less than 2.20
    (B) closest to but not less than 1.20
    (C) closest to but not less than 0.45
    (D) 2.20 or higher

28. For the daily quality control testing, the base-plus-fog level should remain within

    (A) +0.15 of the established levels
    (B) +0.10 of the established levels
    (C) +0.30 of the established levels
    (D) +0.03 of the established levels

29. The screen-cleaning test should be carried out whenever

    (A) there is an upward drift in the operating data levels
    (B) there is a change in the types of chemical used
    (C) there is change in film brand or type
    (D) a mammographer notices dust artifacts on the image

30. Before processing the sensitometric strip each day, the mammographer should

    (A) check the developer temperature
    (B) be sure the view boxes are clean
    (C) clean the cassette screens with screen cleaner
    (D) check the cassettes for dirt or lint

31. The phantom image background optical density should never be

    (A) more than 1.20
    (B) less than 1.20
    (C) more than 1.40
    (D) less than 1.40

32. In the darkroom fog test, the optical density difference between fogged and unfogged areas of the film should NOT exceed

    (A) 1.20
    (B) 0.15
    (C) 0.05
    (D) 0.02

33. In viewing phantom films, which of the following viewing conditions need NOT apply?

    (A) on the same view box
    (B) using the same type magnifier
    (C) at the same time of day
    (D) using the same film emulsion batch

34. In the test for screen contact there were multiple points of small areas (<1 cm in diameter) of poor contact. The corrective action is to

    (A) replace the cassettes; this result is not acceptable
    (B) repeat the test
    (C) return the cassette to clinical use
    (D) clean the screens, wait 15 minutes, then repeat the test

35. One of the two reasons towels are used in the compression test is to

    (A) protect the cassette holder
    (B) ensure that the compression is adequate
    (C) force slower application of compression
    (D) simulate 4 cm of compressed breast

36. For the repeat analysis to be meaningful, a patient volume of at least _____ patients is needed.

    (A) 50
    (B) 100
    (C) 250
    (D) 300

37. Daily processing control can involve all of the following EXCEPT

    (A) cleaning the processor feed tray
    (B) using the sensitometer to measure the densities on the strip
    (C) recording the temperature of the developer tank
    (D) mixing the chemicals

38. Proving that a darkroom fog failure is a result of safelight problems involves

    (A) moving the safe light at least 6 feet from the work surface
    (B) repeating the test with the safe lights off
    (C) checking for light leaks around the doors and passbox
    (D) changing the filter on the safe light

39. The darkroom fog test is performed

    (A) semiannually
    (B) monthly
    (C) weekly
    (D) daily

40. Daily processor control is used to

    1. determine the film speed
    2. check the film contrast
    3. check the stability of the processor

    (A) 1 and 2 only
    (B) 2 and 3 only
    (C) 1 and 3 only
    (D) 1, 2, and 3

41. If, after examining a phantom image, the number of visualized fibers or masses has changed significantly, the next step is to

    (A) record the new values
    (B) call the medical physicist
    (C) call the equipment service personnel
    (D) check the chemistry or temperature then repeat the test

42. Repeated films are

    (A) films used for processor cleaning
    (B) films used for quality control
    (C) films that involve exposure to the patient
    (D) all discarded films

43. If the patient volume at a mammography site is 200 patients per week, the repeat/reject analysis should be done every

    (A) week
    (B) 2 weeks
    (C) 2 months
    (D) 3 months

44. All the fluorescent tubes in the mammography view box should be replaced at the same time because

    (A) fluorescent tubes decrease in brightness with age
    (B) fluorescent tubes will only last about 18–24 months
    (C) they have a higher luminescence than conventional tubes
    (D) it saves time to replace them all at the same time

45. In imaging the phantom, the technical factors used should be the same as those used clinically for a _____ -cm-thick breast of medium glandularity.

    (A) 6.0–6.5
    (B) 5.0–5.5
    (C) 4.0–4.5
    (D) 3.0–3.5

46. Mammography facilities can receive certification from
    1. the ACR
    2. the FDA
    3. an SAC state

    (A) 1 and 2 only
    (B) 2 and 3 only
    (C) 1 and 3 only
    (D) 1, 2, and 3 only

47. An MQSA certificate is issued when a mammography facility has been accredited. This certification is valued for

    (A) 1 year
    (B) 2 years
    (C) 3 years
    (D) 4 years

48. If any of the visual checks fail, the first step is to

    (A) replace the item
    (B) call the medical physicist
    (C) call the processor service
    (D) call the equipment service representative

Answers and Explanations

1. **(B)** The kVp controls the wavelength or the penetrating power of the beam. The kVp will therefore ultimately control the subject contrast, exposure latitude, and image contrast. Remember, however, that as the kVp is reduced, the penetrating ability of the beam is also reduced leading to the use of higher mAs. Higher mAs use increases patient dose. *(Bushong p. 273; Wentz, p. 47)*

2. **(B)** All mammography units are manufactured with tungsten, molybdenum, or rhodium targets matched with the appropriate K-edge filters. These targets have different atomic numbers and therefore different emission spectrums. The characteristic energies of molybdenum are most effective for fatty breast tissue. The characteristic x-rays produced using rhodium targets with rhodium filtration are similar to those from molybdenum but, because rhodium has a slightly higher atomic number, more bremsstrahlung x-rays are produced. However, the energy of the K-characteristic x-rays will be 2–3 keV higher, which provides a better penetration of dense breast although it generally results in lower contrast images. Tungsten targets with tungsten filtration are not used because here bremsstrahlung x-rays will predominate at energies above and below the 17- to 24-keV range. The x-rays most useful in maximizing contrast in breast tissue are in the 17- to 24-keV range. *(Bushong, p. 310; Wentz, p. 47)*

3. **(B)** Mammography uses very low energy x-ray beams and it is important that the x-ray tube window does not attenuate the low-energy photons. The proper filter shapes the emission spectrum of the x-ray beam and makes it compatible with the image receptor and breast characteristics of each patient. In general, mammography units either have borosilicate or beryllium as port windows. *(Bushong, p. 311)*

4. **(D)** The heel of the anode will reduce the intensity of the x-ray beam. In general, the smaller the anode angle, the larger the heel effect because there is increased absorption of the rays (Figure 2–1). *(Bushong, p. 117)*

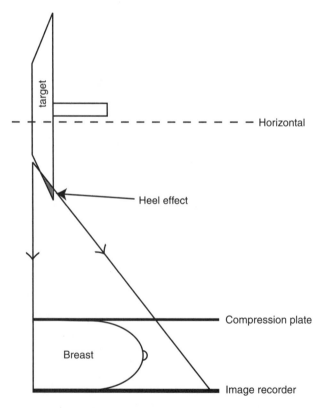

Figure 2–1. Heel effect. The shaded area indicates absorption of x-rays by the target. This results in the lower beam at the anode end of the tube. This effect is minimized in mammography by placing the anode toward the nipple (lower density) area of the breast.

5. **(D)** Both the height and angle of the compression paddle make a difference in the final image. A compression device with a rounded or gently sloping posterior edge does not allow uniform compression of the posterior area of the breast. The height of the compression reduces the chance of chest tissue overlapping on the mammogram. The design of the lip has a lesser effect on the anterior aspect of the breast. *(ACR, pp. 30–33)*

6. **(C)** Compression does all of these, but its *primary* goal is to reduce the breast thickness uniformly—(separate breast structures) and allow uniform penetration by the x-ray beam. *(ACR, pp. 30–33)*

7. **(B)** The most common cause of failure of the AEC is improper placement of the detector. Processing affects the mammographic image after exposure and mammographic quality control ensures correct processing conditions. Decreased radiographic contrast is a result of underexposure, not the cause, and inadequate compression, although it causes uneven densities on the mammogram, does not result from AEC failure. *(ACR, p. 92)*

8. **(A)** The detector system of the AEC allows the unit to respond to different breast composition and various breast sizes. If the detector is placed over fatty breast tissue, the glandular tissue will be underexposed. To produce an adequate exposure, the detector must be placed over the densest or most glandular areas of the compressed breast. *(Andolina, p. 183; Bushong, p. 315)*

9. **(B)** All grids result in increased exposure and patient dose, but improve contrast. The mammography grid, however, has a lower grid ratio than general radiography grids. The grid ratio of mammography grids ranges from 3:1 to 5:1 versus the 6:1 to 16:1 ratio of grids used in general radiography. (Grid ratio = height of the lead strips/the distance between the strips [h/d]). *(Carlton, p. 570; Bushong, p. 310)*

10. **(D)** Higher grid ratios will require too large an increase in exposure. On average, the grids used in mammography range from 3:1 to 5:1, with frequencies of 30–50 lines per centimeter. Typically, a mammography grid may have a grid ratio of 4:1, and although such a grid will double the patient dose when compared to a nongrid exposure, the increased contrast will be significant. *(Bushong, p. 315; Carlton, p. 583)*

11. **(A)** Collimating or decreasing field reduces scatter and therefore improves the contrast. However, because collimating reduces the scattered radiation density to the area, the exposure must be increased. *(Bushong, p. 222; Wentz, pp. 2–23)*

12. **(D)** The compression plate is specifically designed to properly position and compress the breast while reducing discomfort to the patient. The placement of the lip, just beyond the chest wall edge of the image receptor, prevents the projection of an image of the chest wall edge of the paddle on the mammogram. *(AEC, pp. 30–33)*

13. **(A)** The focal spot size is the area that electrons strike on the target. In the design known as the line-focus principle, the target is angled allowing a larger area for the electrons to strike while maintaining a small, effective focal spot. The effective focal spot size is the area projected onto the patient or image receptor. It is also the value quoted when identifying a small or large focal spot. The smaller the target angle, the smaller the focal spot size. Although the resolution and sharpness of the image are directly related to the focal spot size, changes in the SID, OID, and size of the collimated field do not affect the focal spot size. *(Bushong, p. 132; Carlton, p. 402; Wentz, pp. 19–20)*

14. **(B)** Mammography machines generally have two focal spot sizes. The large focal spot may be 0.4 or below (generally 0.3 mm) and the small focal spot ranges from 0.15–0.1 (generally 0.1 mm). Routine work utilizes the large focal spot size. *(Bushong, p. 311)*

15. **(C)** All cassettes are easy to open, durable, and have low absorption characteristics relative to the kVp. Mammography cassettes are designed for use with a single emulsion film and are therefore matched with a single intensifying screen. *(Bushong, p. 316; Wentz, p. 24)*

16. **(C)** An increase in processing time generally increases the developer time with further increase in contrast and film speed. The disadvantage of this system is the increased risk of processing artifacts and the increase in film fog. *(Wentz, pp. 28–29)*

17. **(A)** Digital mammography systems utilize a detector and electronic system instead of a cassette. CAD technology refers to computer-assisted diagnosis, a technology that can be linked to digital systems. Storage phosphors are used with computed radiography systems; the imaging plates or imaging detectors are coated with storage phosphors or photo-stimulatable plates. X-rays will react with the imaging plate to form the latent image (Figure 2–2). *(Bushong, pp. 357–375; Carlton, p. 634)*

18. **(C)** With digital technology, images can be viewed at a workstation. The image at the workstation is called the soft copy image because it can be adjusted for contrast and brightness, or magnified and further enhanced (Figure 2–3). *(Bushong, pp. 357–375; Carlton, p. 635)*

19. **(D)** Despite the numerous advantages of the double emulsion system, these advantages are outweighed by the single largest disadvantage: the system has a lower spatial resolution than the single emulsion system. In double emulsion systems, the emulsions of both screens are activated by the x-rays and will emit light. This crossover light compromises image quality. *(Carlton, p. 587)*

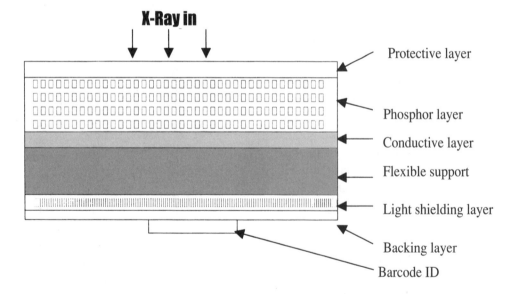

Figure 2–2. A cross-section of an imaging plate. Computer radiography differs from conventional film-screen imaging in the acquisition stage. Instead of a film-screen as the image detector, computer radiography uses a flexible imaging place (IP) coated with storage phosphors or photostimulatable plates. The imaging plates are less than 1 mm thick. They absorb x-ray energy and form a latent image in much the same way a film does. The difference is the wide latitude of the storage phosphors. The higher sensitivity of the imaging plates demonstrates a linear response (input to output) to the intensity of x-ray exposure over a broad range. The IP is constructed much like a conventional screen. Both have a protective laminate to protect the phosphor layer. The IP has a conductive layer to conduct away static; a flexible support layer, which allows IP flexibility; and a backing layer to prevent damage to the IP. The barcode reader on the IP allows for patient information and identification. With such a similar structure, the IP can be placed in modified cassettes and exposed with standard x-ray equipment. The x-ray passes through the patient and reacts with the IP to form the latent image.

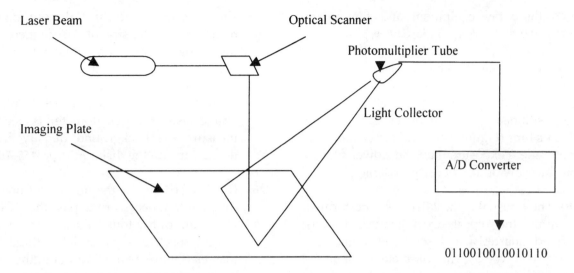

Figure 2–3. A computer reader. To read the latent image, the imaging plate (IP) is inserted into an imaging plate reader or computer reader (CR). The CR reader then scans the image with a laser beam to initiate the emission of light from the storage phosphors. This stored energy leaves the IP in the form of ultraviolet light. The intensity of light emitted from the IP is proportional to the amount of radiation absorbed by the storage phosphor. During the reading process, the light emitted from the IP is collected and sent to a photomultiplier tube. The signal from the tube is amplified and sent to an analog-to-digital converter where it is converted to a digital or electrical signal. The resultant digital information can then be electronically transmitted, manipulated, and stored. The IP can be erased and used again and again by exposing them to strong light.

20. **(B)** The characteristic curve plots the relationship between the optical density of the film and its exposure. The straight-line portion of the curve records the useful range of optical densities. The lowest exposure (base plus fog) is the reading recorded at the toe of the curve, and the highest exposure level is recorded at the shoulder of the curve (Figure 2–4). *(Bushong, p. 256)*

21. **(C)** The characteristic curve is used in quality control to monitor processing conditions by recording changes in the density values. Because of the wide range of variables in x-ray generating equipment, a sensitometer and not the step-wedge is used to produce a uniform optical step wedge on a film, from which the characteristic curve can be plotted. The characteristic curve can interpret characteristics of the film, such as contrast: the steeper the slope the higher the contrast. By plotting the characteristic curves of two films, the speeds of the different films can be compared. A characteristic curve obtained from a step-wedge or penetrometer, however, is capable of monitoring

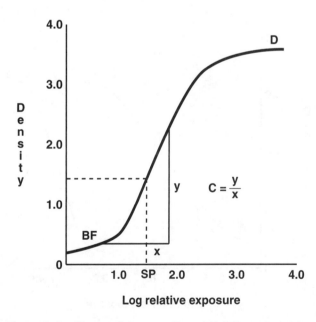

Figure 2–4. Characteristic curve. Normal H & D curve showing base-plus-fog (BF), speed (SP), contrast (C), and maximum density (D) for a single exposure.

both the x-ray equipment and film-screen combination. *(Bushong, p. 256; Carlton, p. 315)*

22. (D) By plotting the characteristic curves of two films the speed of the different films can be compared: the curve of the faster film will be positioned to the left of the curve of the slower film (Figure 2–5). The faster film will require less exposure than the slower film to produce any optical density. *(Bushong, p. 260)*

23. (B) The visual checklist is performed monthly, the repeat/reject analysis is performed quarterly, and screen cleanliness is performed weekly. The complete list of mammography quality control tests and frequency are listed on page 15. *(ACR, p. 119)*

24. (A) The cassette should be loaded with a film for at least 15 minutes before testing to release any trapped air. The air-bleed time refers to the time taken for the air trapped in the cassette to dissipate. *(ACR, p. 141; Wentz, p. 110)*

25. (C) Screen cleanliness requires screen wipes and canned air or a screen cleaner. The densitometer is needed for darkroom fog test to measure the density of the fogged versus the unfogged area of the image. In assessing the screen-film contact, the density at the chest wall area of the wire-mesh image should be between 0.7 and 0.8. In phantom image tests, the densitometer is needed to measure the background density and the density inside the disk. *(ACR, pp. 165–166)*

26. (B) The criteria for the number of objects on the phantom necessary to pass the ACR are a minimum of the four largest fibers, the three largest speck groups, and the three largest masses (Figure 2–6). In addition, the number of test objects of each group type (fibers, specks, and masses) visible in the phantom image should not decrease by more than one-half. *(ACR, p. 268)*

27. (B) In establishing processing controls, decide which sensitometer step has an average density closest to 1.20 (Figure 2–7). This is the *mid-density* (MD) step, sometimes recorded as the *speed index*. Decide which step has a density closest to 2.20, and which step has a density closest to but not less than 0.45. The difference in densities between these two is the *density difference* (DD) or *contrast index*.

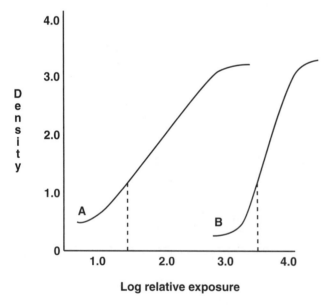

Figure 2–5.   H & D curve-film speed. Graph of H & D curves for two different types of radiographic films. Film A has a faster speed than film B because its speed point is the left of Film B. Film B has a higher contrast than film A because the slope of its curve is steeper than that of Film A.

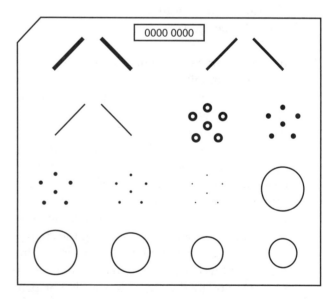

Figure 2–6.   Diagram of phantom. A schematic diagram of the phantom showing the relative position of the different objects embedded within the phantom.

X-Rite®

| 1 |
| 2 |
| 3 |
| 4 |
| 5 |
| 6 |
| 7 |
| 8 |
| 9 |
| 10 |
| 11 |
| 12 |
| 13 |
| 14 |
| 15 |
| 16 |
| 17 |
| 18 |
| 19 |
| 20 |
| 21 |

TIME: DATE: IDNO:

Figure 2–7. Sensitometer strip. The sensitometer will produce a step-wedge pattern of 21 different optical densities. A densitometer is then used to record the base-plus-fog value and the high-, medium-, and low-density measurements. These results are then plotted on the daily processor quality assurance chart.

Suggested performance criteria for the MD and DD are to be within ±0.15 optical density units of the operating level. If the MD or DD exceeds the operating limits by ±0.15, corrective action needs to be taken. Changes in density can be due to chemistry, temperature, replenishment, and so on. *(ACR, pp. 149–164)*

28. **(D)** The base plus fog (B + F) should remain within +0.03 of the operating level. If B + F exceeds the normal level by 0.03, immediate corrective action must be taken. Changes in B + F can be due to chemistry, temperature, replenishment, and so on. *(ACR, pp. 149–164)*

29. **(D)** Although recommended weekly, this test must be carried out whenever dust or any other artifact is seen on the image. Changes in the film brand, processing chemistry, or processing quality control do not affect screen cleanliness. *(ACR, p. 165)*

30. **(A)** The sensitometer strip is used to verify that the processor is operating within normal limits. Of all these answers, only a too high or too low developer temperature will have an impact on the sensitometric strip. *(ACR, pp. 149–164)*

31. **(B)** The background optical density on the phantom should never be less than 1.2 and should not vary by more than ±0.2 (Figure 2–8). The mAs should not vary by more than ±15% from test to test. Optical density should be at least 1.4. *(ACR, pp. 268–269)*

32. **(C)** The optical density difference between the fogged and unfogged areas of phantom

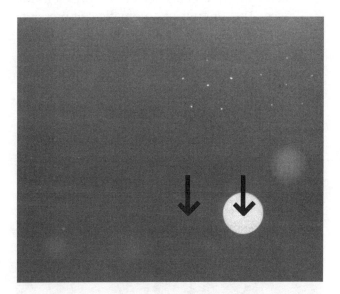

Figure 2-8. Radiograph of phantom. An actual radiograph of a phantom with 1-cm diameter, 4-mm-thick disc. This disc is used for contrast measurement. *Arrows* indicate points where density measurements should be made. The image is scored based on what is seen on the film.

in the darkroom fog test should not exceed 0.05 (Figure 2–9). *(ACR, pp. 189–193)*

33. **(D)** Different individuals will always perceive an image differently. Because of this, the phantom should always be viewed by the same individual, using the same view box and viewing conditions, such as magnification. In addition, the criteria used for viewing the phantom images should be the same as that used when reading mammograms. Because a single film box will not last forever, a new box and therefore a different film emulsion will eventually be necessary. *(ACR, pp. 167–187)*

34. **(C)** Multiple small areas of poor contact (<1 cm in diameter) are acceptable (Figure 2–10). Large areas (>1 cm in diameter) of poor contact, that remain unchanged even after cleaning the cassette, means the cassette fails. *(ACR, pp. 194–198)*

35. **(A)** The towels protect the cassette holder and prevent damage to the compression device. The amount of automatic compression applied is a function of the unit and will not be altered by the presence or absence of a towel. However, the force of the compression device hitting the cassette holder could damage both. *(ACR, pp. 199–201)*

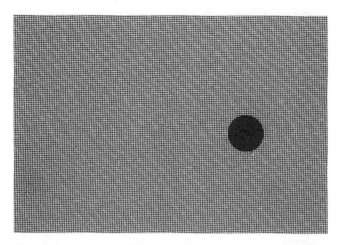

Figure 2–10.   Screen-film contact. A screen should be replaced if it has an area (greater than 1 cm in diameter) of poor contact that cannot be eliminated. Multiple small areas are considered acceptable (sample area shown is 1 cm in diameter).

36. **(C)** The repeat analysis is used to identify problem areas within the department (Figure 2–11). However, for the analysis to be meaningful a sufficient patient volume is needed. The MQSA recommends a meaningful volume of at least 250 patients. *(ACR, pp. 202–203)*

37. **(B)** A sensitometer is designed to expose a uniform optical step wedge onto a film; the densitometer is an instrument that measures the degree of blackening (density) on a film. Daily processings are a means of ensuring that the slight changes in film processing will be corrected before they have an impact on the film artifact, contrast, resolution, and exposure. The developer temperature and the chemistry of the solutions can both impact film contrast. Keeping a clean feed tray reduces film artifacts. *(ACR, p. 339)*

38. **(B)** The simplest way to confirm that the darkroom fog testing failed because of a safelight problem is to repeat the test with the safelight off. If the test passes then the safelight is the problem and the filter could be changed or the light moved to a different location. If the test with the safelight off fails, other areas to check include light leaks around the doors and passbox. *(ACR, p. 192)*

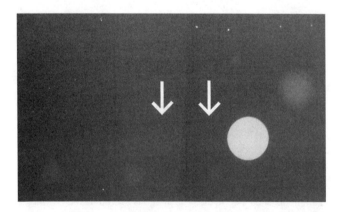

Figure 2–9.   Darkroom fog test. Phantom images showing acceptable levels of darkroom fog. A densitometer is used to measure close to the edge separating the fogged and unfogged portions of the phantom image. The density should not be measured over any test object in the phantom.

Mammography Repeat-reject Analysis   Date From 9/3/01 To 12/28/01

	Projection Repeated Check one for each repeated film						Number of Films	% of Repeats
Reason for Reject	Left CC	Right CC	Left MLO	Right MLO	Left Other	Right Other		
1. Positioning			✓✓	✓✓✓			5	19.2
2. Patient Motion		✓			✓		2	7.7
3. Light Films			✓	✓	✓		3	11.5
4. Dark Films	✓	✓					2	7.7
5. Black Films			✓				1	3.8
6. Static, Artifacts				✓	✓✓		3	11.5
7. Fog		✓	✓				2	7.7
8. Incorrect ID or Double Exposure							0	
9. Equipment Error			✓	✓			2	7.7
10. Technologist Error		✓✓	✓	✓			4	15.4
11. Good Film (No apparent reason)			✓✓				2	7.7

12. Clear Film	6
13. Wire Localization	10
14. Quality Control	7

		Number	Percentage
	Repeats (1-11)	26	1.17
	Rejects (All –1-14)	49	2.21

Total Films Used	2216

Comments	
Action taken	

Figure 2–11. Repeat analysis. A sample of the repeat/reject chart used by technologist to chart the reasons for rejected films. The final percentage of repeats and rejects is calculated as a percentage of the total films used. The percentage of each category of repeated film is calculated as a percentage of the total repeat rate.

39. **(A)** Darkroom fog test is performed semiannually to ensure that the darkroom safelights or other source of light leaks are not fogging the mammographic film. Film fog will result in loss of contrast and therefore loss of diagnostic information. This test should also be performed whenever the safelight bulb or filters are changed. *(ACR, p. 119; Bushong, p. 330)*

40. **(D)** The processor quality control test is used to determine that the processor and processor chemistry are stable and consistent. At the beginning of each day a sensitometric strip is exposed and processed following MQSA guidelines. The medium density evaluates film speed, the density difference evaluates image contrast, and the base-plus-fog value evaluates the level of fog present in the processing chain. By checking and correcting any value that exceeds the normal limits, mammography film will be processed only under optimal conditions to enhance contrast (Figure 2–12). *(ACR, p. 149; Bushong, p. 324)*

41. **(D)** Whenever a test fails, the first corrective action is to verify that the equipment (both the mammographic unit and processor) is operating correctly, and then repeat the test to determine whether the change is real or not. Because the purpose of quality control testing is to ensure optimal conditions before clinical images are processed, significant changes must first be corrected. The medical physicist or the equipment service personnel should be called if the problem cannot be isolated or corrected by the mammographer. *(ACR, p. 186; Bushong, p. 324)*

42. **(C)** Repeated films are those that had to be repeated and resulted in additional exposure to the patient, for example, double exposed films or films with motion. Rejected films are all discarded films, including repeated films. Films used for quality control and processor cleaning are not counted as repeated films. *(ACR, p. 202)*

43. **(D)** Repeat analysis testing is carried out every 3 months (quarterly), unless the patient volume is less than 250 in the quarter. *(ACR, p. 202)*

44. **(A)** Because fluorescent tubes decrease in brightness with age, changing the tubes all at the same time ensures that the mammograms or phantom images are always viewed under identical conditions—uniformity in color and luminance. In addition, it is advisable to replace fluorescent tubes every 18–24 months. *(ACR, p. 209)*

45. **(C)** The mammographic phantom is equivalent to a 4.2-cm-thick compressed breast consisting of 50% glandular and 50% adipose tissue. The technique used should be the same as that used clinically and the film should be processed just like a clinical mammogram. Phantom images are taken to ensure that the optical density contrast and image quality are at optimal levels (Figure 2–13). *(ACR, p. 167; Bushong, p. 325)*

46. **(B)** Under MQSA rules, accreditation and certification are two separate processes. Both are required by the FDA. New rules, effective May 2002, permit certification only by the FDA and SAC states. Accreditation is a process administered by an FDA-approved accreditation body, which can be a private, nonprofit organization or a state agency approved to accredit mammography facilities. In 1997 the FDA approved five accreditation bodies—the American College of Radiology (ACR) and the states of Arkansas, California, Iowa, and Texas. These five bodies all have the authority to implement the MQSA standards through the accreditation process. *(Accreditation and Certification Overview)*

47. **(C)** After completing the accreditation process, the FDA or SAC state will issue a certification that is valid for 3 years and can be renewed as long as the facility remains properly accredited and demonstrates that it meets the MQSA standards during annual inspections. *(Accreditation and Certification Overview)*

48. **(A)** Examples of visual checklist items are a check of mechanical locks or display lighting. Many items are for the mammographer's convenience; some, however, are essential for patient safety and the production of quality images. Missing or broken items should therefore be replaced or repaired immediately. *(ACR, p. 213)*

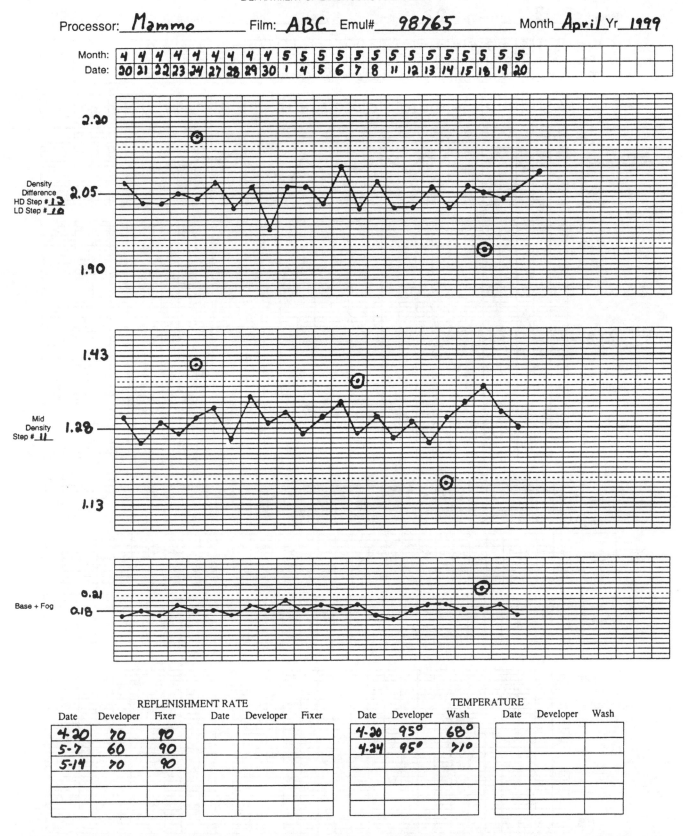

Figure 2–12. Sample processor control chart. The sensitometer strip is exposed and processed each day and the data evaluated and plotted. The result is the processor control chart. Data out of the control limits are circled and the test repeated. The cause of the problem and corrective action is recorded in "remarks" section of the control chart.

(Reprinted with permission of the American College of Radiology, Reston, Virginia. No other representation of this material is authorized without express, written permission from the American College of Radiology.)

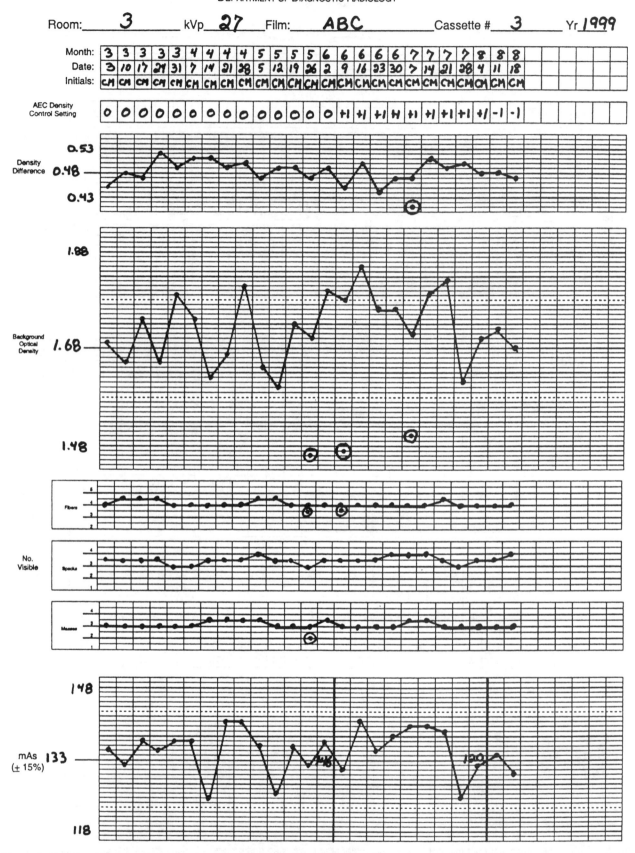

Figure 2–13. Sample phantom control chart. The weekly phantom evaluation checks the film optical density, contrast (density difference), and number of fibers, speck groups, and masses. The results are plotted. Data out of the control limits are circled and the test repeated. The cause of the problem and corrective action is recorded in the remarks section of the control chart.

(Reprinted with permission of the American College of Radiology, Reston, Virginia. No other representation of this material is authorized without express, written permission from the American College of Radiology.)

CHAPTER 3

Anatomy, Physiology, and Pathology of the Breast

Summary of Important Points

LOCALIZATION TERMINOLOGY

The breast is generally described in terms of the face of a clock, and it is also divided into four quadrants.

EXTERNAL ANATOMY

In the female, breasts are accessory glands of the reproductive system with the function of secreting milk for nourishment of the newborn. The female breast is spherical in shape, and size varies with age, menstrual cycle, and lactation. Hormonal stimulation causes the breasts to grow. The breast is loosely attached to the fascia covering the pectoralis major muscle.

The *skin* of the breast, like the skin of the body, is filled with sweat glands, sebaceous glands (oil glands), and hair follicles that open to form the skin pores. The *nipple* lies at the center point of the breast. The *areola* is the smooth, circular darkening surrounding the nipple and contains many small protrusions on its surface (Morgagni's tubercles). The nipple itself contains multiple crevices, within which are 15–20 orifices, or collecting ducts that transfer milk from the lactiferous ducts.

LOCATION

The breasts lie anterior to the pectoralis major. Separating the breast from the pectoral muscle is a layer of adipose tissue and connective fascia referred to as the *retromammary space*.

INTERNAL ANATOMY

The breast is made up of a varying mixture of adipose or fatty tissue, glandular or secretory components, lymphatic vessels, and blood vessels. Cooper's ligaments are the supportive structures of the breast. Fibrous and glandular tissues are usually described together as fibroglandular. The pattern and distribution of the glandular tissue is usually the same bilaterally.

Blood Supply to the Breast

The breast receives its arterial supply from branches of the internal mammary and lateral thoracic arteries. *Veins* that drain the breast form a venous network under the nipple. This network then drains into the axillary and internal mammary veins. Veins are usually larger than arteries and are located more peripherally.

Lymphatic Drainage of the Breast

The primary lymphatic drainage of the breast is to the axilla. The majority of normal axillary lymph nodes are less than 2 cm in size and have a kidney-shaped appearance (Figure 3–1).

HISTOLOGY

The average female breast consists of 15–20 lobes containing numerous glandular lobules held together by connective tissue, blood vessels, and branching ducts (lactiferous ducts). Each of the 15–20 lobes in the breast contains a tree-like pattern of ductal structures radiating out from the nipple.

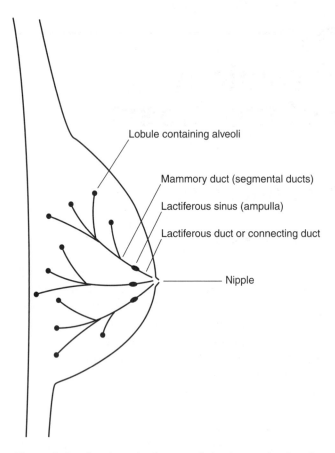

Figure 3–1. A schematic diagram of the breast showing the branching distribution system of a collecting duct. The nomenclature of the duct system is varied.

Lobule containing alveoli

Mammory duct (segmental ducts)

Lactiferous sinus (ampulla)

Lactiferous duct or connecting duct

Nipple

Factors Affecting Tissue Composition

The normal physiologic changes that take place in the breast are related to the onset of menarche, the amount of hormone fluctuation whether normal or synthetic, pregnancy, lactation, and menopause.

MALIGNANT CONDITIONS AND MAMMOGRAPHIC APPEARANCES

Mammographically the breast will be visualized as less dense areas of fat (which appear black on the radiograph) and denser glandular areas (which appear white or gray on the radiograph). Often blood vessels can be seen, especially if they are calcified, and occasionally lymph nodes are visualized within the breast as kidney-shaped oval densities with lucent centers.

The majority of breast diseases occur in the terminal duct lobular units; however, the fibrous or connective tissue can also be involved. Other lesions occur in the larger ducts.

Malignant and benign breast lesions can be placed in five categories:

- Circular/oval lesion may be poorly outlined; circular, oval, or lobulated; and solitary or multiple.
- Spiculate/stellate lesions are radiating structures with ill-defined borders.
- Calcifications may or may not be associated with a tumor.
- Thickened skin syndrome may present over the entire breast and may or may not be associated with an increased density.
- There may be any combination of two or more of the above lesions.

Characteristics of Malignant Circular/Oval Lesions

- High-density—structures such as veins trabeculae cannot be seen through the lesion; for example, invasive ductal carcinoma, sarcoma
- Smooth or lobulated and randomly orientated—not aligned along the trabecular structure of the breast.

Characteristics of Malignant Speculated/Stellate Lesions

- Has a distinct central mass, for example, invasive ductal carcinoma
- Sharp, dense, fine lines of variable length radiating in all directions—the larger the central tumor mass the longer the spicules
- If spicules reach the skin or muscle it may cause localized skin thickening or skin dimpling (retraction)
- Commonly associated with malignant-type calcifications

Characteristics of Malignant Calcification

There are three basic forms of malignant calcifications

- Casting-type calcifications—Fine linear branching calcifications seen on the mammogram as linear, fragmented, or occasionally branching calcifications with irregular contours, for example, ductal carcinoma in situ.

- Granular-type calcifications—Irregular in form, size and density. They resemble granulated sugar or crushed stone. They are usually grouped very close together in single or multiple clusters, for example, ductal carcinoma in situ.
- Powderish calcifications—Multiple clusters of powderish calcifications.

SKIN THICKENING SYNDROME

Skin thickening may be caused by either benign or malignant conditions.

- The skin will appear obviously thickened, generally in the lower dependent portion of the breast.
- The overall density of the breast is increased due to the high fluid content (seen as a course reticular pattern on the mammogram).

BENIGN CONDITIONS AND MAMMOGRAPHIC APPEARANCE

Characteristics of Benign Circular/Oval Lesions

- Radiolucent (e.g., lipoma, oil cyst, galactocele)
- Radiolucent and radiopaque combined (e.g., lymph node, fibroadenolipoma, galactocele, and hematoma).
- Low density (surrounding parenchymal structures can be seen through the lesion; e.g., fibroadenoma, cyst)
- Spherical or ovoid with smooth borders generally aligned in the direction of the nipple along the trabecular structure of the breast.
- Has a halo sign (a narrow radiolucent ring or ring segment around the circumference of the lesion; e.g., cyst).
- Has a capsule (a thin curved radiopaque line surrounding the lesion; e.g., fibroadenoma).

Some exceptions are abscess, hematoma, and sebaceous cyst.

Characteristics of Benign Speculated/Stellate Lesions

- No solid, dense, or distinct central mass
- May have translucent oval or circular area at the center (e.g., radial scar)
- Very fine linear densities or lower density spicules (e.g., radial scars or traumatic fat necrosis)
- Never associated with skin thickening or skin retraction (exception traumatic fat necrosis)

Characteristics of Benign Calcification

- Smooth contours, high uniform density (e.g., plasma cell mastitis)
- Evenly scattered homogenous (e.g., calcified arteries)
- Sharply outlined, spherical, or oval
- Pear-like densities—resemble teacups or pearl drops on the lateral projection (e.g., milk of calcium)
- Bilateral and evenly scattered following the course of the ducts throughout much of the parenchyma
- Ring-like, hollow (e.g., sebaceous gland calcifications)
- Eggshell-like (e.g., oil cyst, papilloma)
- Large size, bizarre shape (e.g., hemangiomas) (Figure 3–2)

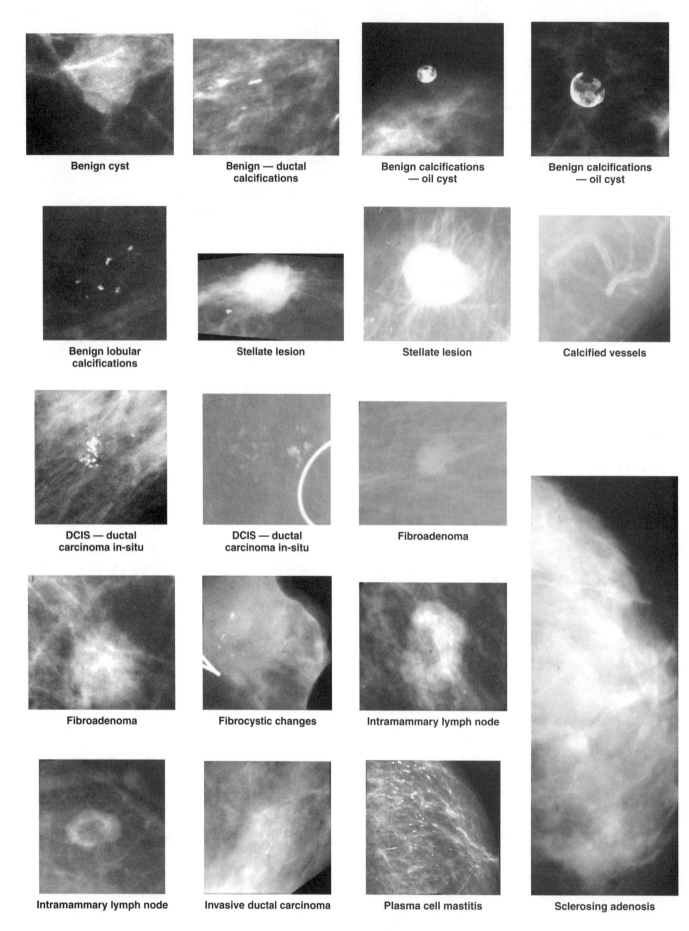

Figure 3–2. Picture summary of breast lesions. (Courtesy of Carol MacKay.)

Questions

1. A lesion located in the upper outer quadrant of the right breast is located in the

   (A) 5:00 o'clock position
   (B) 2:00 o'clock position
   (C) 10:00 o'clock position
   (D) 7:00 o'clock position

2. Morgagni's tubercles are usually found

   (A) on the nipple
   (B) on the lateral border of the breast
   (C) in the terminal duct lobular unit (TDLU)
   (D) on the skin of the areola

3. An inverted nipple

   (A) always indicates breast cancer
   (B) sometimes indicates breast cancer
   (C) never indicates breast cancer
   (D) usually indicates breast cancer

4. Compression of the breast is most effective and most comfortable when applied to the

   (A) medial and lateral aspects
   (B) inferior and superior aspects
   (C) medial and superior aspects
   (D) inferior and lateral aspects

5. The normal breast may have

   (A) 5–10 lobes
   (B) 15–20 lobes
   (C) 25–30 lobes
   (D) 30–40 lobes

6. The structure that gives the breast its support and shape is called

   (A) Montgomery ligament
   (B) Cooper's ligament
   (C) fibroglandular tissue
   (D) fatty tissue

7. The breast extends vertically from the

   (A) 1st through the 9th rib
   (B) 2nd through the 9th rib
   (C) 2nd through the 6th rib
   (D) 3rd through the 10th rib

8. The thickest portion of the breast is the

   (A) areola
   (B) nipple
   (C) tail of Spence
   (D) inframammary crease

9. Cooper's ligaments attach anteriorly to the

   (A) deep fascia of the lobes
   (B) fascia of the skin
   (C) posterior surface of the breast
   (D) connective and supporting stroma

10. Fatty tissue is generally _____ and on the mammogram is seen as areas of _____ optical density.

    (A) radiolucent/lower
    (B) radiopaque/higher
    (C) radiolucent/higher
    (D) radiopaque/lower

11. Typically, a patient with dense fibrous and glandular tissue throughout the entire breast is

   (A) age 20 or younger
   (B) age 50 or older
   (C) over age 70
   (D) under age 45

12. Glandular tissue is usually found in the _____ of the breast.

   (A) medial and lower inner quadrant
   (B) central and upper outer quadrant
   (C) medial and lower outer quadrant
   (D) upper inner quadrant and central

13. Lymph drainage from the medial half of the breast is generally directed to the

   (A) internal mammary lymph nodes
   (B) external mammary lymph nodes
   (C) axillary lymph nodes
   (D) axilla

14. Immediately behind the nipple the connecting duct widens to form the

   (A) lactiferous sinus
   (B) ampulla acinus
   (C) TDLU
   (D) segmental duct

15. The portion of the breast that holds the milk-producing element is the

   (A) ampulla
   (B) segmental duct
   (C) lobule
   (D) lactiferous sinus

16. Veins are normally located

   (A) in the periphery of the breast
   (B) central areas of the breast
   (C) in the axilla area of the breast
   (D) in the medial areas of the breast

17. The terminal ductal lobular unit consists of the

   (A) mammary ducts and the extralobular terminal ducts
   (B) intralobular terminal duct and the segmental ducts
   (C) the extralobular terminal ducts and the lactiferous ducts
   (D) both the extralobular and the intralobular terminal ducts

18. A patient began taking synthetic hormones 6 months prior to her current mammogram. The mammogram is most likely to

   (A) be unchanged from the previous year
   (B) show increased glandular tissue compared to her previous mammogram
   (C) show decreased glandular tissue compared to her previous mammogram
   (D) show increased fatty tissue compared to her previous mammogram

19. The mammogram shows that the patient's breast consists primarily of adipose tissue. This patient is most likely to be

   (A) on hormone therapy
   (B) over age 60
   (C) under age 20
   (D) over age 35

20. A patient is to have a routine baseline mammogram, but it is determined that the woman is lactating. What should be done?

   (A) Lactating breasts are extremely sensitive; the mammogram should be postponed.
   (B) The mammogram should be done; the radiation has no effect on lactation.
   (C) Although lactating breasts are extremely dense, the mammogram should not be rescheduled.
   (D) Lactation causes increased glandularity; the mammogram should be postponed.

21. The craniocaudad mammograms of the same woman prior to menopause and 1 year after the onset of menopause are compared. The woman has never taken synthetic hormones. What is the most likely difference?

(A) The mammogram taken prior to menopause shows signs of atrophy.

(B) The mammogram taken after the onset of menopause shows signs of atrophy.

(C) There will be little or no change in the glandularity of the breast.

(D) The mammogram taken after menopause will show increased glandularity.

22. Which of the following will affect the ratio of glandular tissue to total breast tissue?

1. the woman's genetic predisposition
2. ratio of total body adipose tissue to total body weight
3. drastic weight gain or weight loss

(A) 1 only

(B) 1 and 2 only

(C) 2 and 3 only

(D) 1, 2, and 3

23. What procedure should be followed if a symptomatic patient who is lactating is scheduled for a mammogram?

(A) The mammographer should attempt spot compression views only.

(B) The mammogram should be done, but the study may be limited.

(C) Lactating breasts are extremely dense; the mammogram should be postponed.

(D) Lactation causes increased glandularity; the mammogram should be postponed.

24. A woman is referred to as nulliparous. This means

(A) she has never given birth to a child

(B) the woman has had one child

(C) the woman has never produced a viable offspring

(D) she carried a pregnancy to a point of viability regardless of the outcome

25. An asymptomatic patient presents with an oval, lobulated tumor with unsharp margins. There is no evidence of a halo sign.

(A) If the lesion is also radiolucent it is likely to be benign.

(B) The lesion could be malignant.

(C) All oval lesions are benign.

(D) The absence of a halo indicates malignancy schematic.

26. The tumor seen in Figure 3–3 indicates

(A) invasive ductal breast carcinoma

(B) a mammographically malignant tumor

(C) a mammographically benign tumor

(D) a low-density tumor typical of benign lesions

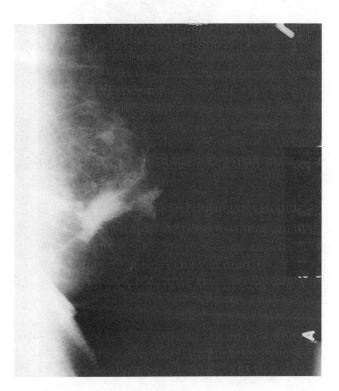

Figure 3–3.

27. The calcifications seen in Figure 3–4 have the typical appearance of

   (A) mammographically malignant-type calcifications
   (B) mammographically benign-type calcifications
   (C) calcifications typical of an oil cyst
   (D) calcified microhematomas

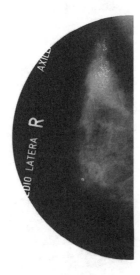

Figure 3-4.

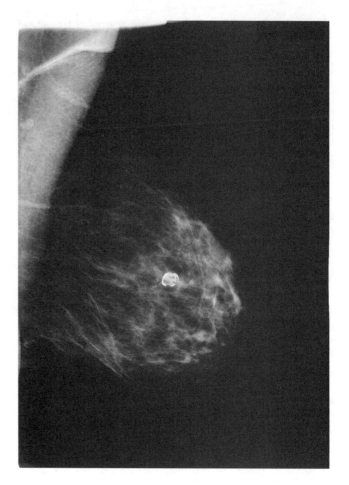

Figure 3–5.

28. Characteristics of a malignant stellate tumor include which of the following?

   1. the spicules are generally bunched together
   2. the presence of a central tumor mass
   3. the larger the tumor, the longer the spicules

   (A) 1 only
   (B) 1 and 2 only
   (C) 2 and 3 only
   (D) 1 and 3 only

29. The calcifications seen in Figure 3–5 have the typical appearance of

   (A) an oil cyst
   (B) plasma cell mastitis calcification
   (C) a small hematoma
   (D) a calcified sebaceous gland

30. Sclerosing duct hyperplasia

   1. can sometimes be mistaken for carcinoma
   2. sometimes has a solid dense central tumor
   3. is usually not associated with skin thickening or dimpling over the lesion

   (A) 1 only
   (B) 1 and 2 only
   (C) 2 and 3 only
   (D) 1 and 3 only

31. A mammogram shows a low-density radiopaque tumor. It is oval, lobulated, and a halo is seen along one border only. The next step should be

(A) pneumocystogram

(B) ultrasound

(C) biopsy

(D) no further testing; the tumor is benign

32. A galactocele

(A) is generally large

(B) is usually associated with trauma

(C) is associated with nursing

(D) usually has irregular borders

33. A lipoma

(A) is generally seen as a high-density radiopaque lesion on the mammogram

(B) can be a huge encapsulated lesion occupying the entire breast

(C) may have irregular borders typical of malignant lesions

(D) is usually difficult to image mammographically

Answers and Explanations

1. **(C)** Each breast can be divided into four quadrants: the upper outer quadrant (UOQ), upper inner quadrant (UIQ), lower outer quadrant (LOQ), and lower inner quadrant (LIQ). The exact locations within the quadrant are represented by viewing each breast (separately) as a clock face (Figure 3–6). Lesions can also be described in relation to the nipple (e.g., subareola or below the nipple). *(Wentz, p. 57)*

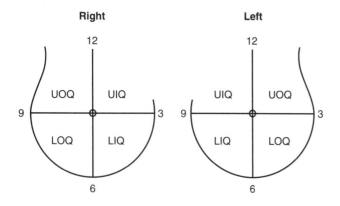

Figure 3–6. Breast localization pictures. The breast can be viewed in different ways: (1) As a clock with clock-time descriptions within the breast. (2) Using the four-quadrants method: the upper-outer quadrant (UOQ), the upper-inner quadrant (OIQ), the lower-outer quadrant (LOQ), and the lower-inner quadrant (LIQ). Note that the four o'clock position on the right breast represents the LIQ but on the left breast would indicate the LOQ.

2. **(D)** Morgagni's tubercles are elevations formed by the opening of the ducts of the Montgomery's glands, specialized sebaceous-type glands found on the areola, not the nipple. *(Wentz, p. 11)*

3. **(B)** The normal nipple can be either flattened or inverted, both unilaterally and bilaterally. However, a nipple that suddenly becomes inverted or flattened can indicate malignancy. *(Logan-Young, p. 16; Wentz, p. 11)*

4. **(D)** The breast is most secured at the superior and medial aspects. The lateral borders of the breast and the inferior aspect (inframammary crease) are the most mobile portions. Compression is most effective when applied to the mobile aspects of the breast. *(Wentz, p. 45)*

5. **(B)** On average, a breast has 15 lobes. The number can, however, be as low as 10 or as high as 20. *(Harris, p. 4; Wentz, p. 13)*

6. **(B)** Cooper's ligaments are a network of fibrous and elastic membranes. They incompletely sheath the lobes of the breast. The ligaments start at the most posterior portion (base) of the breast and extend outward to attach to the anterior superficial fascia of the skin. Fibroglandular and fatty tissue make up the breast parenchyma. The Montgomery is a gland, not a ligament. *(Harris, p. 4; Wentz, p. 13)*

7. **(C)** The breast extends vertically from the clavicle (the second or third rib) to meet the abdominal wall at the level of the sixth or seventh rib and horizontally from the midsternum to the midaxillary line (the latissimus dorsi muscle). *(Harris, p. 3; Wentz, p. 11)*

8. **(C)** The upper outer quadrant, which extends toward the axilla, is known as the axillary tail or the tail of Spence. It is the thickest portion of the breast. Thorough knowledge of the anatomic extent of the breast is critical in breast imaging. *(Logan-Young, p. 16)*

9. **(B)** Cooper's ligaments are strands of connective tissue that run between the skin and deep fascia to support the lobes of the breast. They start at the most posterior portion (base) of the breast, extend outward, and attach to the anterior fascia of the skin. *(Wentz, p. 13)*

10. **(C)** Fatty tissue is radiolucent and will therefore show as higher optical density areas on mammograms (white or gray). Fibrous and glandular tissue are less radiolucent and will show as lower optical density on the mammograms (black). *(Wentz, p. 12)*

11. **(D)** In general, the amount of fat and glandular tissue varies with age. Glandular tissue predominates in younger women, whereas fatty tissue predominates in older patients. A patient under 20 is unlikely to have regular mammograms. *(Logan-Young, p. 15; Wentz, p. 13)*

12. **(B)** The majority of glandular tissue is distributed in the breast bilaterally and is located centrally and laterally toward the upper outer quadrant, extending toward the axilla. Most breast cancer arises from the glandular tissue. *(Logan-Young, p. 17; Wentz, p. 13)*

13. **(A)** The main direction of drainage from the lateral half of the breast tends to be into the pectoral group of axillary lymph nodes and from the medial half of the breast into the internal mammary lymph nodes. *(Wentz, p. 13)*

14. **(A)** From the nipple orifice a connecting or lactiferous duct immediately widens into the lactiferous sinus (or ampulla). The ampulla is a pouch-like structure that holds milk (when it is being produced). The ampulla then narrows to become the segmental or mammary ducts. These branch into smaller ducts with decreasing diameter until becoming a lobule. *(Logan-Young, p. 15; Thomas, p. 1069)*

15. **(C)** From the nipple, the mammary ducts become smaller and smaller until becoming a lobule. The lobule is also called the terminal ductal lobular unit (TDLU). The TDLU is lined with a single layer of epithelial cells and a peripheral layer of myoepithelial cells

and consists of both the extralobular and the intralobular terminal ducts. The intralobular terminal ducts (ITD) hold the alveolar glands, which are the milk-producing elements of the breast. *(Logan-Young, p. 15)*

16. **(A)** Veins are larger than arteries. Unlike arteries, they are normally located peripherally and easily seen. Mammographically they appear as low-density, radiopaque vessels. Both arteries and veins can be outlined by calcifications. *(Andolina, p. 171; Wentz, p. 13)*

17. **(D)** The TDLUs are further divided into the extralobular terminal duct (ETD), which is a small duct leading into the terminal ductules, and the intralobular terminal duct (ITD), located at the end of the terminal ductules. The ETD is surrounded by elastic tissue and lined by columnar cells. The ITD has no surrounding elastic tissue and contains cuboidal cells (Figure 3–7). The ITD holds the milk-produc-

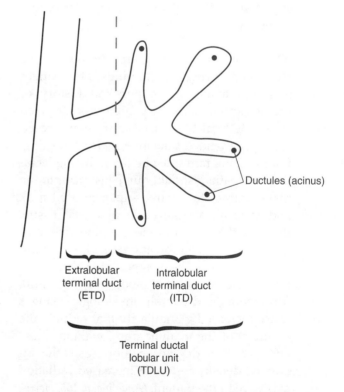

Figure 3–7. Picture of TDLU. The TDLU increase and decrease in size and number depending on menstrual cycle, pregnancy, lactation, and hormone use. The TDLU are responsible for milk production and it is here that most cancers originate. The ductal system ends at the terminal ductal lobular unit (TDLU). The unit is further divided into extralobular terminal unit (ETD) and intralobular terminal unit (ITD).

ing elements of the breast, called the ductules or acinus (plural, acini). Each lobule can have 10–100 terminal ductules. *(Harris, p. 4; Wentz, p. 12)*

18. **(B)** Increased or decreased glandularity of the breast is a part of the normal physiologic changes that take place. It can be related to menarche, hormonal fluctuation whether normal or synthetic, pregnancy, lactation, or menopause. The two most prominent hormones active in pathology are estrogen (responsible for ductal proliferation) and progesterone (responsible for lobular proliferation and growth). *(Logan-Young, p. 15; Wentz, p. 12)*

19. **(B)** Patients over age 60 will most likely have fatty breast; glandular tissues predominate in young women and adipose tissue (fat) predominate in older women. Patients under 20 usually have dense breast, but are also less likely to have a mammogram. Hormone therapy is likely to increase the glandular nature of the breast. *(Logan-Young, p. 15)*

20. **(D)** Ideally, a mammogram should not be scheduled during lactation unless the patient is symptomatic, has a personal history of breast cancer, or is very high risk. In such cases, the total time of lactation may exceed the recommended time interval for screening. If a mammogram must be done during lactation, the patient should nurse just prior to the mammogram to remove superimposed milk and improve visualization of breast tissue. Because this is a routine baseline mammogram on an asymptomatic patient, the mammogram should be postponed. During lactation the increased blood supply, milk production, and overall physiologic changes cause increased glandularity that reduces the accuracy of the mammogram, making it less effective as a diagnostic tool. Also, the increased density results in increased radiation exposure to the patient. *(Andolina, p. 153; Harris, pp. 11–12; Wentz, p. 12)*

21. **(B)** Generally, atrophy of mammary structures begins at menopause and ends 3–5 years later. After menopause, the breast loses its supportive tissue to fat, producing a smaller breast, or a larger, more pendulous one. This process is called involution. *(Harris, p. 12; Wentz, p. 12)*

22. **(D)** The total amount of glandular tissue increases and decreases with hormonal fluctuations, use of synthetic hormones, and menopause. The amount of glandular tissue versus fatty tissue will also depend on a woman's genetic predisposition. It is therefore possible to find young women with fatty breast and older women with extremely dense, glandular breast. Weight gain and loss also increase or decrease the fat content of the breast tissue, thereby affecting the overall glandularity of the breast. *(Logan-Young, p. 15; Wentz, p. 12)*

23. **(B)** Ideally, a mammogram should not be scheduled during lactation unless the patient is *symptomatic*, has a personal history of breast cancer, or is very high risk. In such cases the total time of lactation may exceed the recommended time interval for screening. If any of the above reasons apply and if a mammogram must be done during lactation, the patient should nurse just prior to the mammogram to remove superimposed milk and improve visualization of breast tissue. During lactation the increased blood supply, milk production, and overall physiologic changes cause increased glandularity that reduces the accuracy of the mammogram, making it less effective as a diagnostic tool. Also, the increased density results in increased radiation exposure to the patient. *(Andolina, p. 153; Harris, pp. 11–12; Wentz, p. 12)*

24. **(A)** A nulliparous is the condition of not having given birth to a child. Parity is the terminology used if a woman carries a pregnancy to a point of viability (20 weeks of gestation) regardless of the outcome. Other terminology is multiparity, regarded as having borne more than one child, and primapara, a woman who has delivered a child of 500 g (or of 20 weeks' gestation) regardless of its viability. *(Thomas, pp. 1243, 1317, 1415)*

25. **(B)** Although a halo is typically present in benign lesions, absence of a halo does not necessarily prove malignancy. However, any circumscribed radiopaque tumor with unsharp borders and no demonstrable halo sign should lead to suspicion of malignancy, regardless of density (Figure 3–8). *(Tabár, p. 52)*

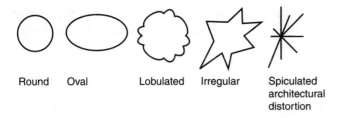

Round   Oval   Lobulated   Irregular   Spiculated architectural distortion

Figure 3–8. Breast masses. The borders or shape of breast masses may be round, oval, lobulated, irregular, or spiculated. A spiculated border is a strong indication for malignancy, whereas a smooth border is a strong indication for a benign abnormality. These, however, are indicators and will not necessarily determine the presence or absence of carcinoma.

26. **(B)** The mammogram shows a stellate tumor; the nipple and areola are retracted. The skin is thickened over the lower and outer portions of the breast. Although the mammogram can suggest carcinoma and may be highly suspicious for carcinoma, only a microscopic diagnosis (histology analysis) reveals the exact type. The presence of a central tumor mass with associated spicules is typical of malignant stellate tumors. The spicules are dense and sharp, radiate from the tumor surface, and usually are not bunched together. When they extend to the skin or areolar region, they cause retraction and local thickening. Generally, the larger the tumor, the longer the spicules. *(Tabár, p. 97)*

27. **(A)** These calcifications are typical of mammographically malignant-type casting and granular microcalcifications. Casting calcifications are produced when carcinoma in situ fills the ducts and their branches. The shape of the cast is determined by the uneven production of calcifications and the irregular necrosis of the cellular content. The contours of the cast are always irregular in density, size, and length and the casts are always fragmented. A calcification is seen as branching when it extends into adjacent ducts. Also, the width of the ducts determines the width of the castings. Granular type calcifications are seen as mammographically similar in appearance to granulated sugar or crushed stones. These are also malignant-type calcifications. Oil cysts are generally seen mammographically as eggshell-like calcifications and a microhematoma is a mixed-density oval or circular calcification. *(Tabár, p. 154)*

28. **(C)** A typical malignant stellate tumor has a central tumor with dense spicules radiating in all directions. The spicules are separate and increase in length with increased tumor size. If the spicules reach the skin, there is localized dimpling or skin thickening. *(Tabár, p. 94)*

29. **(A)** This calcification has the typical appearance of an oil cyst. Oil cysts are generally seen mammographically as egg-shell like calcifications. Plasma cell mastitis calcifications follow the course of the ducts. Some may be elongated and branching, some needle-like, and some ring-like or oval, but all are sharply outlined, high density, and have smooth borders. If they are periductal, they have central lucencies. Calcified sebaceous glands are typically ring-like oval calcifications with lucent centers; there are two types, depending on where the calcifications started. Calcifications within a sebaceous gland are hollow or ring-like calcifications; calcifications within the cavity are punctate calcifications. A microhematoma is a mixed-density oval or circular calcification. *(Tabár, pp. 199, 208)*

30. **(D)** Radial scar or sclerosing duct hyperplasia is benign and rarely palpable. It is often mistaken for carcinoma and its exact nature is the subject of some controversy among pathologists. Generally, the radial scar has no central tumor. There can be translucent, oval, or circular areas at the center of the lesion and the lesion's appearance varies from one mammography projection to another. Regardless of the size of the lesion, there is gen-

erally no associated skin thickening or dimpling and no discernible palpable mass. *(Tabár, pp. 95–96)*

31. **(B)** A partial halo around a lesion suggests a mammographically benign tumor. An ultrasound would be the best next step to differentiate solid versus a cyst. After the ultrasound a pneumocystogram could be used to assess the inside margins of the tumor. *(Tabár, p. 37)*

32. **(C)** A galactocele is a benign, milk-filled cyst with a high fat content. These lesions are gen-erally associated with lactation. They are usually circular, with sharply defined borders and have densities that are a combination of radiolucent and radiopaque. They are often left alone, but if painful they can be drained using needle puncture. Often they yield a yellow fluid. *(Tabár, p. 26)*

33. **(B)** A lipoma is a fatty tumor. It is radiolucent and may be huge, occupying the entire breast. It is easily seen mammographically and is not metastatic. *(Tabár, p. 21; Thomas, pp. 1118–1119)*

CHAPTER 4

Mammographic Technique and Image Evaluation

Summary of Important Points

BREAST COMPRESSION

Before applying compression, the mammographer should consider the natural mobility of the breast. The breast is easier to compress from the inferior and lateral aspects. The initial automatic compression should never exceed 45 pounds (200 Newtons) of pressure; the patient should not be in pain, but the breast must be taut to fingertip contact.

Compression

- reduces dose to the breast by reducing tissue thickness.
- brings lesions closer to the film for more accuracy when evaluating size.
- decreases motion unsharpness because the breast is immobilized.
- increases contrast, reducing the amount of scattered radiation by decreasing thickness.
- separates superimposed areas of glandular tissue; compression spreads apart overlapping tissue, reducing confusion caused by superimposition shadows, and allowing visualization of the borders of circumscribed lesions.
- allows a more uniform density by flattening the base of the breast to the same degree as the more anterior regions, permitting optimal exposure of the entire breast in one image.

MAGNIFICATION

Magnification is ideal in imaging small areas, such as areas of suspicious microcalcifications or lesions, specimen radiographs, or at surgical sites. Unfortunately, the use of magnification increases patient dose because the breast is placed much closer to the source of radiation.

- A grid is not necessary with magnification.
- A small focal spot must be used with magnification.

SELECTION OF TECHNICAL FACTORS

- The kVp selection or penetrating power of the beam will influence the subject contrast and exposure latitude, and therefore the image contrast. Consideration should also be given to the patient's breast tissue structure. Too high kVp will result in loss of contrast (image too dark or gray). Too low kVp will be high contrast in the medium-density range but result in loss of detail visibility in the dense breast tissue.
- For a given kVp, increasing the mAs alters the optical density of the final mammogram. In general, increasing the mAs increases the mA but not the exposure time.
- The *reciprocity law* states that the density produced on the radiograph is equal to any combination of mA and exposure time as long as the product of mAs is equal. However, the reciprocity law fails at long and short exposures because the film is exposed to light from the intensifying screens. With long and short exposures, reduced film speed and an increase in exposure factors are required. Most modern AEC systems provide automatic correction for film reciprocity failure. If necessary, using a higher kVp, varying the target and/or filtration material, or using a faster screen-film combination will correct reciprocity failure. Also, the length of the exposure time must always be considered because of the possibility of motion unsharpness.

• When using AEC, the position of the detector varies depending on breast size and tissue composition.

EVALUATION OF IMAGE QUALITY

Positioning

The routine series for breast imaging is the CC and the MLO. The CC projection should always demonstrate as much medial tissue as possible because this area is most likely to be missed on the MLO. The MLO will visualize the maximum amount of breast tissue if the angle used is parallel to the pectoral muscle.

Compression

Improperly compressed breast tissue will result in overlapping tissue structures, nonuniform exposure (especially of the denser breast tissue), overpenetration of the thinner breast tissue, poor penetration of the thicker portion, and motion unsharpness.

Exposure

With adequate exposure, it is difficult to see the skin and subcutaneous tissue until the images are masked to block out extraneous viewbox light. Areas of the film with optical densities below 1.0 are generally underexposed. The densest area on the film is the area of pectoralis muscle and it is the only area that should have an optical density below 1.0.

Contrast

In breast tissue, contrast is usually highest in thinner breast and lowest in thicker breast due to more scattered radiation and greater tissue absorption of low kVp radiation in the thicker breast. Without contrast, breast parenchyma with different tissue densities will have very similar optical densities.

Sharpness

The ability of the mammographic system to capture fine details in the image is defined as *sharpness*. If the image is not sharp, it is referred to as *unsharp*. Unsharpness may be the result of motion blur, poor screen-film contrast, characteristics of the screen (faster screen results in more unsharpness), geometric unsharpness (due to large focal spot size, increase in OID, or decrease in SID), or due to the use of double emulsion systems.

Noise

The decreased ability to see tiny structures, such as calcifications on the image, defines noise. The major cause of noise is scatter and quantum mottle, that is, fluctuation in the number of x-ray photons forming the image. The use of high mAs, low kVp, and slower image receptors reduces quantum mottle.

Artifacts

Any variation of density on the image that is not a reflection of the attenuation differences in the subject can be considered artifacts. Examples of artifacts are pick-off, scratches, fingerprints, dirt, lint, or dust.

Collimation

In mammography, collimation is to the image recorder and not to the breast.

Labeling

Standardized labeling in mammography is important because mammograms can be legal documents and it is important that the films are not misinterpreted. In the final rules of the MQSA, labeling is divided into required, highly recommended, and recommended.

Questions

1. Which of the following statements is (are) true?

   1. Compression increases image sharpness by reducing the focal spot size
   2. Compression increases contrast by reducing the thickness of the penetrated tissue
   3. Compression increases the uniformity of the image making diagnosis easier

   (A) 1 only
   (B) 1 and 2 only
   (C) 2 and 3 only
   (D) 1, 2, and 3

2. The compression force should not exceed _____ on the initial power drive (automatic) mode

   (A) 25 lbs
   (B) 35 lbs
   (C) 40 lbs
   (D) 45 lbs

3. In assessing the degree of compression for any one patient the mammographer should take into consideration

   1. the maximum to which the patient's breast can actually be compressed
   2. the amount of compression the patient can tolerate
   3. compression that should be just sufficient to immobilize the breast

   (A) 1 only
   (B) 1 and 2 only
   (C) 1 and 3 only
   (D) 2 and 3 only

4. Manual compression in mammography

   (A) must be between 25 and 45 lb
   (B) depends solely on breast size
   (C) depends on breast size and the patient's pain tolerance
   (D) generally depends on the patient's pain tolerance

5. Some considerations that could be given to women with painful breasts include

   1. having the patient take ibuprofen prior to the mammogram
   2. scheduling the mammogram just after the menstrual cycle
   3. explaining, before the examination, the importance of compression

   (A) 1 only
   (B) 1 and 2
   (C) 2 and 3
   (D) 1, 2, and 3

6. Compression will do all of the following EXCEPT

   (A) bring tissue closer to the image receptor
   (B) reduce patient dose
   (C) improve image contrast
   (D) decrease spatial resolution

7. Compression reduces radiation to the breast by

   (A) providing a uniform breast thickness
   (B) decreasing breast thickness
   (C) decreasing motion unsharpness
   (D) separating superimposed areas of glandular tissue

8. What principle does compression use to visualize the borders of circumscribed lesions?

    1. It brings the lesion closer to the film
    2. It spreads apart overlapping tissue
    3. It separates superimposed areas of glandular tissue

    (A) 1 only
    (B) 1 and 2 only
    (C) 2 and 3 only
    (D) 1, 2, and 3

9. Ideally, compression should be accompanied by

    1. a thorough explanation to increase patient cooperation
    2. arrested inspiration to reduce motion
    3. an explanation of the dosage to reduce fear of radiation

    (A) 1 and 2 only
    (B) 2 and 3 only
    (C) 1 and 3 only
    (D) 1, 2, and 3

10. Patients who are allowed to play an active role in applying the compression are usually

    1. less likely to tolerate the compression
    2. more likely to tolerate the compression
    3. more relaxed during the compression

    (A) 1 only
    (B) 2 only
    (C) 1 and 3 only
    (D) 2 and 3 only

11. Magnification can be used to assess the

    (A) margins of a lesion
    (B) size of a lesion
    (C) location of a lesion
    (D) density of a lesion

12. With calcifications, magnification can be used to assess

    1. the number
    2. morphology
    3. distribution

    (A) 1 only
    (B) 1 and 2 only
    (C) 2 and 3 only
    (D) 1, 2, and 3

13. In general, greater magnification will require the use of a

    (A) larger focal spot size
    (B) smaller OID
    (C) smaller focal spot
    (D) larger SID

14. A grid is not necessary during magnification because

    (A) grid use decreases spatial resolution
    (B) the greater the magnification the smaller the focal spot
    (C) the large OID produces the same effect as a grid
    (D) magnification will magnify the normally invisible grid line

15. The air gap in magnification increases contrast by

    (A) magnifying detail
    (B) reducing scatter
    (C) clarifying borders of masses
    (D) improving visualization

16. If the magnification view is performed without using a small focal spot, the resulting image will be magnified

    (A) and blurred
    (B) and sharply outlined
    (C) with increased contrast
    (D) with increased detail

17. The greater the magnification factor the greater the

1. skin dose
2. focal spot size
3. scatter

   (A) 1 only
   (B) 2 only
   (C) 1 and 2 only
   (D) 2 and 3 only

18. Magnification is beneficial in all of the following situations EXCEPT

   (A) surgical site of a patient with a lumpectomy
   (B) imaging a specimen radiograph
   (C) evaluating microcalcifications in a lesion
   (D) routine imaging

19. Using a small focal spot size is recommended for magnification

   (A) to reduce the resultant loss of image detail
   (B) because of increased patient dose
   (C) to compensate for the small OID
   (D) to compensate for motion unsharpness

20. The greatest disadvantage of magnification is

   (A) increased OID
   (B) increased patient dose
   (C) decreased contrast
   (D) increased risk of motion unsharpness

21. Optical densities below 1.0 in the dense glandular tissue is considered

   (A) underexposed
   (B) overexposed
   (C) normal exposure
   (D) above average but not overexposure

22. Some causes of underexposure include

1. processing deficiencies
2. inadequate compression
3. improper AEC setting

   (A) 1 only
   (B) 1 and 2 only
   (C) 2 and 3 only
   (D) 1, 2, and 3

23. Inadequate automatic exposure compensation can cause

   (A) underexposed films
   (B) overexposed films
   (C) normal exposure films
   (D) above average but not overexposed films

24. The leading cause of false-negative mammograms in dense breast tissue is

   (A) motion
   (B) overexposure
   (C) underexposure
   (D) grid lines

25. Overexposure is sometimes called the recoverable error because

   (A) it can be corrected during developing
   (B) high illumination and masking can overcome it
   (C) magnification can overcome it
   (D) the use of small focal spot sizes will reduce it

26. Increased kVp during mammography is sometimes necessary to penetrate dense fibroglandular tissue. Increased kVp, however, generally causes

   (A) increased contrast
   (B) decreased contrast
   (C) motion unsharpness
   (D) less scatter

27. Rhodium is not used as the primary anode material because

    (A) rhodium has an emission spectrum similar to tungsten
    (B) the higher energy of the rhodium beam is unsuitable for small breast
    (C) the lower energy of the rhodium beam is unsuitable for small breast
    (D) rhodium anodes are more expensive

28. If the backup time stops a breast exposure the radiographer should repeat the radiograph using a

    (A) higher kVp setting
    (B) greater density compensation
    (C) higher mAs setting
    (D) different AEC setting

29. The type of x-rays created from displacement of K-shell binding electrons in the molybdenum atom are called

    (A) photoelectric
    (B) characteristic
    (C) Compton
    (D) bremsstrahlung

30. The function of the filter in mammography is to remove

    1. low-energy x-rays not needed to produce the breast image
    2. high-energy x-rays that cause a reduction of contrast
    3. low energy x-rays that increase patient dose

        (A) 1 only
        (B) 2 and 3 only
        (C) 1 and 3 only
        (D) 1, 2, and 3

31. If the AEC cell is placed over an area of adipose tissue on a breast with a mixture of adipose and glandular tissue, the areas of glandular tissue will be

    (A) underexposed
    (B) overexposed
    (C) normally exposed
    (D) the AEC cell position will not affect the exposure

32. Causes of poor contrast include all of the following EXCEPT

    (A) inadequate exposure
    (B) lower kVp
    (C) inadequate compression
    (D) failure to use a grid

33. The use of low kVp and high mAs will serve to

    (A) reduce noise and increase contrast
    (B) reduce contrast and reduce noise
    (C) increase noise and reduce contrast
    (D) increase contrast and increase noise

34. A highly recommended labeling that is not required by the MQSA is

    (A) technologist identification
    (B) date stickers
    (C) technical factors
    (D) flash card identification system

35. Lack of breast compression is most likely to cause
    (A) geometric unsharpness
    (B) screen unsharpness
    (C) motion unsharpness
    (D) parallax unsharpness

36. Increasing the kVp by 2 points will

    (A) force a doubling of exposure time
    (B) reduce the exposure time by half
    (C) have no effect on the exposure time
    (D) increase the contrast

37. The technologist can differentiate motion unsharpness from screen unsharpness because

    (A) motion unsharpness is generally localized to a small area

    (B) screen unsharpness is generally localized to a small area

    (C) motion unsharpness will result in blurring

    (D) screen unsharpness is less likely at exposures below 2 seconds

38. Increasing the kVp will increase the

    1. optical density on the image

    2. penetrating power of the beam

    3. subject contrast and exposure latitude

        (A) 1 and 2 only

        (B) 2 and 3 only

        (C) 1 and 3 only

        (D) 1, 2, and 3

Answers and Explanations

1. **(C)** Compression makes the breast tissue more uniform and reduces the thickness through which the x-ray beam must pass. This produces uniform densities that are easier to interpret. Although compression increases image sharpness, compression has no impact on the focal spot size. *(ACR, p. 199)*

2. **(D)** According to the MQSA guidelines, the compression force for the initial power drive must be between 111 and 200 Newtons (15 and 45 lbs) and should not exceed 45 lbs. Too little compression will compromise the image; too much can damage breast tissue. *(ACR, pp. 200–201)*

3. **(B)** Ideally, compression should be applied until the breast tissue is taut. But if the patient is in pain at maximum compression, this will be a disincentive to return for annual mammograms. The patient will generally be able to tolerate more compression if they are prepared for it, and if it is applied slowly. Although compression immobilizes the breast and reduces motion, compression just adequate to immobilize the breast is usually insufficient to separate breast tissue. *(ACR, pp. 30–33)*

4. **(C)** The initial compression in mammography should be between 25 and 45 lbs in the automatic mode. In general, the amount of manual compression depends on the patient's breast size and patient's tolerance for compression. Some patients may require more manual compression to adequately compress the breast. *(ACR, p. 199; Wentz, p. 105)*

5. **(D)** Often the patient will be able to tolerate more compression if the need for compression is explained to the patient. Patients with particularly sensitive breasts will benefit from pain medication prior to the mammogram. Also, the breast is often more sensitive to pain just before or during the menstrual period. *(ACR, p. 33)*

6. **(D)** The spatial resolution or image blur defines the detail, accuracy, and clarity of an image. Compression increases spatial resolution by reducing patient thickness; the tissue is therefore closer to the image receptor. The tissue is thinner; there is therefore less scatter and the contrast is improved. Less radiation dose is used to penetrate the thinner breast tissue. *(Bushong, pp. 210–211)*

7. **(B)** Although the primary goal of compression is to decrease motion unsharpness by immobilizing the breast, compression also reduces radiation dose to the breast by decreasing the thickness through which the radiation must pass, thus allowing less exposure. *(Andolina, p. 58; Bushong, p. 314)*

8. **(D)** Compression spreads overlapping tissue and separates superimposed areas of glandular tissue. This allows visualization of the borders of lesions. *(Andolina, p. 58; Bushong, p. 314)*

9. **(C)** Often, the patient is able to tolerate more compression if the need for compression is explained. Knowledge of the procedure generally alleviates fears, especially fears of the unknown. Any explanation should include

an explanation on dosage. Throughout the examination, the patient should be encouraged to relax. Having the patient take a deep breath prior to holding the breath during the exposure is generally contraindicated. The patient may alter her position as the lungs expand, and the expanding ribs and lungs generally contract the pectoral muscles increasing discomfort during the mammogram. The patient should be simply advised to 'stop breathing' without moving her body or first taking a deep breath. *(Andolina, pp. 10, 33–34)*

10. **(D)** Studies have shown that if a patient plays an active role in applying the compression that the patient will be able to tolerate the compression better and will be more relaxed during the compression. The more the patient knows about compression and the more the patient understands the more she will be relaxed. To give the patient an active role in compression, the mammographer can allow the patient to apply the compression or constantly monitor the patient, stopping the compression when the patient indicates. *(Wentz, p. 44)*

11. **(A)** Magnification cannot be used to assess lesion size because it gives a magnified view. Location and density are also not assessed using magnification because magnification does not include the entire breast. Magnification is, however, capable of providing views that can assess the lesion's margins. *(ACR, pp. 59–60)*

12. **(D)** *Morphology* is the form or structure of the calcification. By magnifying the area of interest, magnification provides views that can be used to assess the number, distribution, and morphology of the calcifications. *(ACR, pp. 59–60)*

13. **(C)** As the magnification factor increases, the focal spot must be reduced or the thickness of the part decreased to maintain sharp images. Both of these factors are used in magnification. *(Andolina, p. 64; Bushong pp. 264–265)*

14. **(C)** The large OID or air gap acts like a grid in reducing the amount of scattered radiation

reaching the film. Grid use in magnification increases exposure times, increasing tube loading, and thus increasing motion artifact due to long exposure times. Radiation dose to the patient is also increased. *(Andolina, p. 63)*

15. **(B)** The large air gap acts like a grid and reduces scatter, thus improving contrast. Positioning the breast away from the film takes advantage of the inverse-square law: the intensity of the scattered radiation is reduced because the distance between the film and the object is increased. *(ACR, pp. 59–60)*

16. **(A)** Whenever the relationship between the source, object, and image are altered, as in magnification, there is an increase in focal spot blur. To keep focal spot blur at a minimum and to compensate for the reduced resolution during magnification, a small focal spot must be used. *(Andolina, p. 63; Bushong, p. 268; Wentz, p. 23)*

17. **(A)** Radiation intensity is related to the square of the distance; therefore, as the patient is moved closer to the x-ray tube, patient dose increases. Thus, the greater the magnification factor the greater the skin dose. Also, as the magnification factor increases, a small focal spot must be used to maintain a sharp image. Scatter is insignificant during magnification because of the air gap. *(Bushong, pp. 303–304; Wentz, p. 23)*

18. **(D)** Magnification is ideal for imaging small areas such as the surgical site of a patient with a lumpectomy, specimen radiography, or microcalcifications. With magnification, microcalcifications that would otherwise be missed can be seen. Magnification should not be used in routine imaging because the entire breast may not be imaged, and patient dose is increased. *(Bushong, p. 316; Wentz, p. 23)*

19. **(A)** The focal spot blur (*penumbra* or *geometric unsharpness* are the old terms) is caused by a large effective focal spot. Whenever the relationship between the source, object, and image is altered, as in magnification, there is an increase in focal spot blur. To keep focal spot blur at a minimum, a small focal spot is

used. Remember, a small focal spot necessitates a lower mA output and thus results in increased exposure time and risk of motion. *(Bushong, p. 268)*

20. **(B)** Unfortunately, magnification increases patient dose. Using a magnification factor of 1.4 may actually double the radiation dose to the patient because the breast is placed closer to the radiation source. *(Bushong, p. 268)*

21. **(A)** Normally, optical densities on the mammogram are in the 1.6 or higher range. The trend clinically is to have higher optical densities to adequately penetrate the glandular tissue and produce higher-contrast images. *(ACR, p. 92; Andolina, p. 92)*

22. **(D)** All cause a reduction in the density of the image, which causes a film to appear underexposed. If the developer temperature decreases, the film speed decreases, resulting in lower film density. Poor compression causes uneven densities, leading to underpenetration of portions of the breast. Improper selection of the AEC results in inadequate x-ray penetration of the glandular tissue of the breast. *(ACR, p. 97; Andolina, pp. 75, 98, 184)*

23. **(A)** The AEC produces a diagnostic density determined by the tissue placed directly over the AEC cells. If the AEC compensation is inadequate, then the backup time is reached because the selected kVp is too low to penetrate the breast tissue. The result is a light film. *(ACR, p. 97; Carlton, p. 573)*

24. **(C)** Underexposure of dense breast tissue is the leading cause of false-negative mammograms. If the area is underexposed calcifications or even subtle density differences are not detected in the glandular breast tissue. *(ACR, p. 97)*

25. **(B)** Overexposure can be overcome by using high illumination and masking. Modern automatic processing makes correcting techniques during developing unworkable and adjusting the focal spot size or magnification will not correct for overexposure. Underexposure is an unrecoverable error in that lost contrast cannot be restored in light areas of the film. The film has to be repeated with greater film exposure. Note that extreme overexposure decreases contrast. *(ACR, p. 98)*

26. **(B)** The kilovoltage primarily influences the quality of the x-ray beam. As the kVp increases, the penetrating quality of the beam increases—more x-rays pass through the breast and reach the film at higher kVp. There is, therefore, less differential absorption and thus a reduction in subject contrast. *(Bushong, p. 273)*

27. **(B)** Rhodium targets with rhodium filters have an emission spectrum similar to molybdenum, not tungsten. However, because rhodium has a higher atomic number, a rhodium emission spectrum has a slightly higher K-edge and more bremsstrahlung x-rays than the emission spectrum for a molybdenum target tube filtered with molybdenum, which shows almost no bremsstrahlung x-rays and has lower K-edge x-rays. Bremsstrahlung x-rays are produced more easily in target atoms with a high atomic number. The significance of this in mammography is that the keV energy of the rhodium is designed to penetrate thicker, more dense breast tissue. *(Bushong, p. 310; Carlton, p. 581)*

28. **(A)** The backup timer in newer mammography units delivers a test exposure to check for adequate penetration. The density compensation circuit and the mAs should not be increased; because the primary reason for backup time is that the beam has low-energy photons that are unable to penetrate the breast. Increasing the compensation circuit does not increase the energy of the beam. Each step on the compensation circuit generally results in a 12–15% change in mAs. Increasing the mAs increases the overall film density, but similar to the compensation circuit, this does not increase the penetrating power of the beam. Selecting another AEC setting may result in an underpenetrated image if the new AEC setting is placed over a less dense area of the breast. *(Carlton, p. 574)*

29. (B) The molybdenum anode will produce x-ray photons with energies in the range of 17–20 keV. The most prominent of these x-ray photons are characteristic and will account for 30% of the total x-rays in the molybdenum beam at 30 kVp. The emission spectrum shows almost no bremsstrahlung x-rays because bremsstrahlung x-rays are produced more easily in target atoms with high atomic numbers, such as tungsten. *(Bushong, p. 310; Carlton, p. 580)*

30. (D) Filtration must be used at the tube port window on all mammography machines. It is important that the x-ray tube window not filter out any of the useful energy beam. The filter must be the same element as the x-ray tube target to allow the K-characteristic x-rays to expose the breast while stopping the lower or higher bremsstrahlung x-rays. Most mammography tubes have an inherent filtration of 0.1 mm Al. The total filtration cannot be less than the equivalent of 0.5 mm Al. *(Bushong, p. 312; Carlton, p. 581)*

31. (A) The AEC detects the beam after the x-ray passes through the breast. Because the AEC stops the exposure when it estimates that the correct exposure is reached, positioning the AEC over fatty breast tissue stops the exposure before there is sufficient exposure to penetrate the denser tissue. *(ACR, p. 97; Carlton, p. 573)*

32. (B) Excessive and not lower kVp will cause poor contrast, although some mammographic film now allows significantly higher kVp without sacrificing image contrast. Low contrast mammograms will have a uniform appearance making it difficult to differentiate between different breast tissue thicknesses. Other causes of poor contrast include processing deficiencies, use of low contrast film, improper target material, and/or filtration. *(ACR, pp. 100–101)*

33. (A) Contrast is the ability to see subtle density differences and will be higher at lower kVp, where there is great tissue absorption and less scattered radiation. Noise defines the ability to see minute structures on the image. Reducing noise involves reducing the scattered radiation and quantum mottle.

Noise is therefore lowest at low kVp and high mAs. *(ACR, pp. 100, 105; Bushong, p. 273)*

34. (D) The labeling guidelines under MQSA rules is divided into three areas: required, strongly recommended, and recommended. The flash card patient identification system is strongly recommended because it is the most permanent and will be reproduced on a copy, unlike the stick-on labels. Recommended labeling are date stickers, technical factors (kVp, mAs, exposure time, and target-filter), force of compression, compressed breast thickness, and the degree of obliquity. Required ladeling is:

- Name of patient and additional patient identifier
- Date of examination
- View and laterality (placed near the axilla using the standardized codes approved by the FDA)
- Facility name and location, including the city, state, and zip code
- Technologist identification
- Cassette/screen identification
- Mammography unit identification—if there is more than one unit

(ACR, pp. 26–27)

35. (C) Sharpness is the ability to see fine detail on the mammography image, and patient motion is the most common form of unsharpness. Motion blurring is common with exposure above 2 seconds and can be prevented by proper communication. Good compression will reduce breast thickness, therefore allowing shorter exposure times. Screen unsharpness is a result of poor screen–film contact and can be caused by air trapped between the film and the screen during loading. Geometric unsharpness is caused by increase in focal spot size or OID or by a decrease in SID. Parallax unsharpness results from the use of double emulsion films and is generally not a factor in mammography imaging. *(ACR, p. 102)*

36. (B) The kVp can have a major impact on the exposure time and the dose. As the kVp is increased, the exposure time decreases rapidly—50% for every 2-point drop in kVp. The dose will also decrease by 15 to 20% for a 2-point drop in kVp because a higher kVp setting will allow the use of lower mAs and therefore lower patient doses. As the kVp increases, however, there is less differential absorption leading to a reduction in subject contrast. *(ACR, p. 101; Bushong, p. 273)*

37. **(B)** In screen unsharpness there is a further spread of light from the screen before it reaches the film. This type of unsharpness is independent of the exposure time; unlike motion unsharpness, which covers a wider area, unsharpness due to poor screen contact is usually localized. All unsharp images are referred to as blurry. *(ACR, pp. 104–105)*

38. **(B)** The kVp controls the wavelength or penetrating power of the beam. Increasing the kVp influences the subject contrast and exposure latitude, therefore affecting the image contrast. The main factor influencing the optical density is the mAs. Increasing the mAs will increase the quantity of the electron beam. *(Bushong, p. 273; Wentz, p. 47)*

CHAPTER 5

Positioning and Interventional Procedures

Summary of Important Points

STANDARD PROJECTIONS

Craniocaudal

- Make the exposure on suspended respiration.
- Position the film tray at the level of the inframammary crease when the breast is elevated.
- Position the patient's head away from the side being examined.
- Position the patient's feet apart with weight equally distributed.
- Position the patient's arm closest to breast being examined by the patient's side. Position the other arm raised and holding the machine for support.
- Dense areas of the breast should be adequately penetrated.
- The nipple should be in profile and centered on the film.
- The medial and lateral aspects of the breast must be included in the collimated area. (The pectoralis major muscle is seen approximately 20% of the time.)
- The craniocaudal (CC) projection (Figure 5–1) should include, within 1 cm, the amount of tissue measured on the mediolateral oblique (MLO) film.
- Appropriate markers and labeling must be used as required by the ACR.

Mediolateral Oblique

- Make the exposure on suspended respiration.
- The degree of tube angulation will vary between 30 and 70 degrees depending on patient size; thin patients require steeper angulation than heavier patients.
- Drape the arm closest to the breast being imaged over the top of image recorder. Place the upper border of the image recorder in the armpit.

- Compression must adequately support the anterior breast tissue to prevent sagging and distortion of the ductal architecture. As compression is applied, use one hand to support the anterior breast tissue to avoid skin folds. Use other hand to adjust the skin over the sternum and clavicle to reduce the "pulling sensation."
- The pectoral muscles should be demonstrated to level of the nipple.
- Appropriate markers and labeling must be used as required by the ACR.
- Common problems with the MLO view are
  - drooping breast
  - abdominal tissue does not permit proper compression and positioning of the patient
  - the posterior portion of the breast is not imaged (the inframammary fold is not visualized)

ADDITIONAL POSITIONS/PROJECTIONS

Supplemental projections become useful when the standard views selected are inadequate. Sometimes patient history or body build is such that the standard projections are difficult to obtain. Other reasons to take additional films include the following:

- A suspicious area is seen in one of the routine views but not on the second projection.
- Additional views may allow the patient to avoid the trauma of having an invasive procedure such as needle localization (e.g., a spot film may prove an area of suspicious density to be overlapping tissues).

Exaggerated Craniocaudal (XCCL)

- To image lesions in the lateral aspect of breast not seen on the CC view

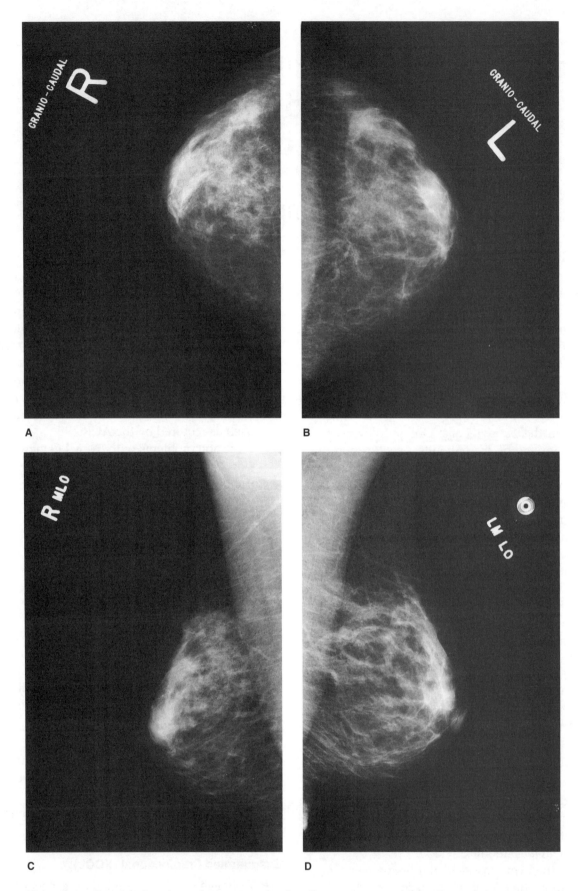

Figure 5–1. Complete four-view series mammogram. A routine mammogram showing the normal appearance of (A) RCC, (B) LCC, (C) RMLO, and (D) LMLO.

Mediolateral 90° (ML)

- To verify a finding or localize a lesion in another dimension (necessary during needle localizations)
- To locate a lesion not seen on a CC projection if lesion is seen only on the MLO projection
  - medial lesions move up on the lateral from their position on the MLO
  - lateral lesions move down on the lateral from their position on the MLO
  - central lesions do not move significantly from the MLO to the ML
- To prove benign breast calcifications (e.g., "teacup"-type calcifications are seen on the ML only)

Caudocranial or From Below (FB)

- To image small breast
- Used on kyphotic patients
- Used on patients with pacemakers
- To better visualize lesions in the superior or upper quadrants of the breast

Lateromedial (LM)

- To improve detail of a lesion located in the medial aspect of the breast
- To perform preoperative localization of an inferior and/or lateral lesion
- May be more comfortable for some patients

Axillary Tail (AT)

- Formerly known as the Cleopatra view
- To visualize the tail of the breast

Cleavage (CV) or "Valley View"

- To show lesions deep and medial to the chest wall (medial breast tissue)

Tangential Projection (TAN)

- To demonstrate a view of the area in question without superimposition of breast tissue
- Often used to locate skin calcification or lesions thought to be near the skin; sometimes a lead spot marker is placed over the area of interest during the exposure

Lateromedial Oblique (LMO)

- Used when the standard MLO projection is difficult to obtain because of patient body build

- Used when patients have a pacemaker
- Used with patients with chest surgery
- Used when patients have a prominent sternum
- Used to evaluate the medial aspect of the breast

MODIFICATIONS

Magnification (M)

- To improve imaging of fine detail, especially when analyzing calcifications
- Magnification must be done only on the smallest focal spot and with the correct magnification devices
- Magnification does not use a grid because of the increased OID

Rolled Lateral (RL) or Rolled Medial (RM)

- The breast is rolled laterally or medially.
- This view is useful in removing superimposed tissue when imaging dense breast (the lesion is "rolled" off or away from the dense tissue).

Rolled Superior (RS) or Rolled Inferior (RI)

- The breast is rolled superiorly or inferiorly.
- This view is useful in removing superimposed tissue when imaging dense breast (the lesion is "rolled" off or away from the dense tissue).

SPECIAL SITUATIONS

Breast Implants (ID Technique)

The standard series of views for a patient with an implant are the routine CC and MLO views plus modified compression views. Most implants can be displaced by modified compression views (implant-displaced or ID views)

Standard views are taken to demonstrate the posterior breast tissue surrounding the margins of the implant. Compression is used for immobilization only. Do not compress the implant.

The modified compression technique requires pulling the natural breast tissue forward while simultaneously pushing the implant back toward the chest wall. Compression is therefore applied only to the breast tissue. Modified views are done in the CC, MLO, and sometimes the ML projection (Figure 5–2).

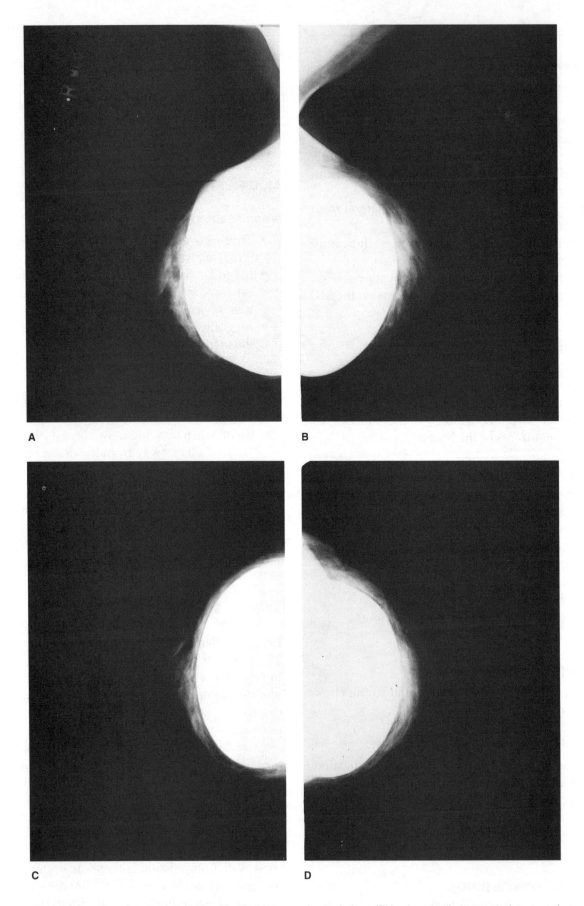

A

B

C

D

Figure 5–2. Complete implant series. Modified compression technique (Eklund method) demonstrating normal (A–D) and modified compression (E–H).

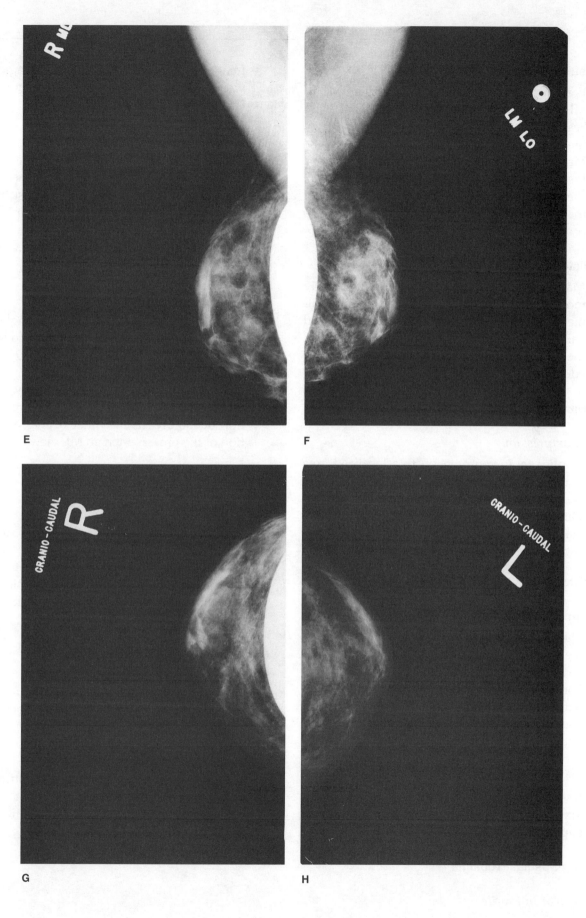

Figure 5–2. *(continued)*

Postsurgical Breast

- For a lumpectomy patient, a CC and an ML or MLO are usually taken of the surgical site.
- Scar markers are useful to identify the site of the surgical scar.
- Magnification views may be required.
- Postmastectomy imaging is controversial. Views may include the CC or a spot view of the area of concern, and an AT view or MLO projection.

Irradiated Breast

- Mammograms should be performed 6–12 months after completion of radiation treatment. Earlier mammograms are of limited value because of prominent residual changes, including parenchymal stromal and dermal edema.

Localization of Suspected Abnormalities

Spot Compression

- Applies more compression to a localized area of interest using a smaller compression paddle
- Helps to evaluate a suspicious area
- Can be performed in any projection or with magnification

IMAGING PHYSICALLY IMPAIRED PATIENTS

Patient on a Stretcher

- The CC can be done with patient recumbent on the stretcher and turned on alternate sides. The x-ray tube is rotated 90°.
- For the MLO, the tube is positioned at 0°. The patient is rolled onto the side being examined and the image receptor positioned under the patient's breast.

Patient in a Wheelchair

- Use the FB view if possible
- Try using wheelchairs with removable arm support

Solving Special Problems

Nipple Not in Profile

- Always image the entire breast first.

- Image the nipple separately, taking nipple views with the nipple in profile.
- Use nipple markers only if necessary.

Skin Folds or Wrinkling of the Breast

- Use an index finger to smooth out the breast as you compress.
- Sometimes, to avoid skin folds, breast tissue is eliminated from the original radiograph.
- If breast tissue is eliminated on the original radiograph, always take additional views to supplement the original.

Patients With Uneven Breast Thickness

- Reevaluate the patient—check the angle of the image receptor (it should be parallel to the pectoral muscle)/height of image receptor.
- If it is impossible to compress the lower half of the breast on the MLO position, two views may be necessary: one of the AT (upper portion of the breast) the other of the lower portion of the breast (often an ML view).

Patients With Difficult Body Habitus

Thin Patients

- Use manual technique if the breast does not cover the first photocell.
- To help bring the pectoral muscle onto the image receptor, roll the patient to the side being examined, bringing the elbow of side under consideration forward.

Patients With an Extremely Obese Upper Arm

- Tape "fat roll" out of position or manipulate the extra tissue from the upper arm behind the image receptor.
- Use sectional imaging with extremely large patients.
- Care should be taken to image the entire breast (the breast tissue must overlap).
- Label the films for proper evaluation (e.g., MLO upper or MLO lower).

SPECIMEN RADIOGRAPHY

The specimen is the breast tissue sample removed during a biopsy. A radiograph of the specimen is necessary to ensure the area under suspicion is totally removed and the margins are clean. In imaging the specimen,

- speed and efficiency are important because the patient may be under anesthesia.
- always use compression.
- magnification may help to visualize microcalcifications.
- a grid is not usually necessary.

INTERVENTIONAL PROCEDURES

Ductography
Ductography is used on patients with abnormal nipple discharge. The lactiferous duct is cannulated. A small amount of contrast media is injected into the ducts. Radiographs are taken in the CC and ML (90°) positions. The purpose of the examination is to determine the location and number of lesions. The examination does not determine if the lesion is malignant or benign.

Pneumocystography
When a patient develops a breast cyst, it may be necessary to evaluate the cyst for debris or abnormal growth. The cyst is aspirated and air is injected to evaluate the inner wall of the cyst. This procedure may also be done under ultrasound guidance.

Ultrasound
Ultrasound is not a screening tool, but it is an important adjunct to mammography. Ultrasound can be used to determine if a mass is solid or fluid filled, during needle-guided excision biopsy, cyst aspiration, or core-needle biopsy. Ultrasound is also useful to assess implants to detect leaks.

Cyst Aspiration/Pneumocystography
Cyst aspiration/pneumocystography is performed either under mammographic or ultrasound guidance. In cyst aspiration, the cyst is drained or emptied using a needle. Once the cyst has been aspirated, a pneumocystograph can be performed. Here, air is injected into the cyst to outline the inner walls.

Stereostatic Localization
Stereostatic localization uses computerized stereo equipment to take core or fine-needle aspiration (FNA) samples. The computer calculates the proper coordinates of the lesion in the breast and enables placement of the needle in the exact location of the lesion.

Preoperative Needle Localization
Nonpalpable abnormalities (lesions or microcalcifications) cannot be felt; therefore, the lesion must be localized to a specific area to minimize the amount of tissue that will be removed surgically.

Fine Needle Aspiration
Cellular material is removed from the area in question for cytologic analysis, possibly reducing the necessity for a surgical breast biopsy. The accuracy of FNA is dependent on the individual performing the procedure (radiologist, cytologist, or surgeon).

Core Biopsy
With core biopsy, a larger sample of tissue is obtained than with FNA. Tissue samples are obtained with an 11- to 14-gauge needle and sent for histologic analysis. There are a number of commercial modifications of the basic core biopsy principle that provide state-of-the-art alternatives to open surgical biopsies. These include the Minimally Invasive Breast Biopsy (MIBB), Vacuum-assisted Core Biopsy (VACB), and Advanced Breast Biopsy Instrumentation (ABBI).

Questions

1. Which projection is used to determine if a lesion is medial or lateral to the nipple?

    (A) CC
    (B) MLO
    (C) TAN
    (D) ML

2. If any breast tissue is missed on the MLO projection it is likely to be

    (A) medial breast tissue
    (B) lateral breast tissue
    (C) inferior breast tissue
    (D) superior breast tissue

3. The posterior nipple line (PNL), visualized on the ML, should be within how many centimeters of the PNL on the CC?

    (A) 0.25
    (B) 0.50
    (C) 1.00
    (D) 1.50

4. Which of the following conditions must be met when imaging the breast in the MLO?

    1. The pectoral muscle should extend to or below the PNL.
    2. Visualized fat should be posterior to all the fibroglandular tissues.
    3. The inframammary fold should be open.

        (A) 1 and 2 only
        (B) 2 and 3 only
        (C) 1 and 3 only
        (D) 1, 2, and 3

5. In positioning for the CC projection, if the C-arm of the mammography unit is raised too high the inframammary fold is over elevated, resulting in loss of

    1. superior breast tissue
    2. inferior breast tissue
    3. posterior breast tissue

        (A) 1 and 2 only
        (B) 2 and 3 only
        (C) 1 and 3 only
        (D) 1, 2, and 3

6. The single view that will best visualize the maximum amount of breast tissue is the

    (A) CC
    (B) MLO
    (C) ML
    (D) XCCL

7. In general, the tube is angled between 30 and 70° when imaging patients in the MLO position. For tall, thin patients the angulation is about

    (A) 30–40°
    (B) 40–50°
    (C) 50–60°
    (D) 60–70°

8. The position used to determine whether an abnormality is superior or inferior to the nipple is the

    (A) CC
    (B) MLO
    (C) XCCL
    (D) TAN

9. The principle of mobile versus fixed tissue is used in mammography imaging to image the maximum

    (A) medial breast on the MLO projection
    (B) inferior breast on the CC projection
    (C) superior breast on the MLO projection
    (D) medial tissue on the CC projection

10. In the CC projection of the breast the image receptor is positioned

    (A) at the level of the inframammary crease
    (B) below the level of the inframammary crease
    (C) at the level of the 7th rib
    (D) just medial to the zyphoid process

11. In positioning for the MLO the tube is always angled

    (A) 90°
    (B) 60°
    (C) 50°
    (D) none of the above

12. What projection/position is shown in Figure 5–3?

    (A) CC
    (B) MLO
    (C) CV
    (D) XCCL

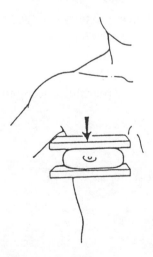

Figure 5–3. (© 2000 The American Registry of Radiologic Technologists.)

13. When positioning for the right CC, where should the patient place the left arm?

    (A) bring backward, to remove the shoulders from the imaging area
    (B) bring forward so the patient can hold the handle bar
    (C) bring forward so the patient can hold the cassette holder
    (D) it should remain at the patient's side

14. Your patient has had recent chest surgery and has a scarred and painful area running along the sternum. With the medial aspect of the breast immobile, which of the following is an alternative to the RMLO?

    (A) RLMO
    (B) LMLO
    (C) RLM
    (D) LML

15. Which projection is best used to visualize the tail of the breast?

    (A) LMO
    (B) TAN
    (C) LM
    (D) AT

16. Calcifications seen on the mammogram are suspected to be in the skin. The best projection necessary to prove this theory is the

    (A) LMO
    (B) TAN
    (C) LM
    (D) AT

17. The projection best used to demonstrate the true representation of medial breast structures in relation to the nipple is the

    (A) LM
    (B) AT
    (C) ML
    (D) TAN

18. A lesion on the lateral aspect of the breast is not seen on the CC. An additional view used to image the lesion could be the

    (A) CV
    (B) XCCL
    (C) FB
    (D) TAN

19. Which projection can be used instead of the CC to image patients with severe kyphosis?

    (A) ML
    (B) TAN
    (C) FB
    (D) CV

20. A lesion moved up on the ML projection from its original position on the MLO. The location of the lesion within the breast is

    (A) laterally
    (B) medially
    (C) inferiorly
    (D) superiorly

21. Which projection is used to prove breast calcifications are benign (teacup type)?

    (A) CC
    (B) XCCL
    (C) FB
    (D) ML

22. Which projection is used to give a tangential view of the area in question without superimposition of breast tissue?

    (A) CV
    (B) TAN
    (C) LMO
    (D) AT

23. Identify the position/projection shown in Figure 5–4.

    (A) FB
    (B) XCCL
    (C) ML
    (D) AT

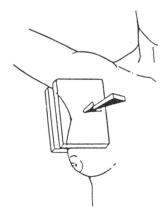

Figure 5–4. (© 2000 The American Registry of Radiologic Technologists.)

24. A barrel-chested patient whose chest wall protrudes outward may have breast tissue extending laterally under the arm. What projection, used to image the breast with the beam directed superiorly to inferiorly, should be taken in addition to the CC?

    (A) AT
    (B) XCCL
    (C) CV
    (D) MLO

25. The FB projection can be useful in imaging

    1. nonconforming patients
    2. abnormalities high on the chest wall
    3. patient with subpectoral implants

    (A) 1 and 2 only
    (B) 2 and 3 only
    (C) 1 and 3 only
    (D) 1, 2, and 3

26. Identify the projection shown in Figure 5–5.

    (A) MLO
    (B) CV
    (C) LM
    (D) ML

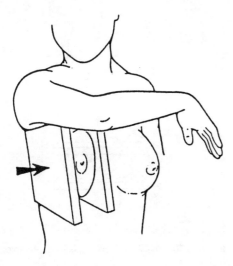

Figure 5–5. (© 2000 The American Registry of Radiologic Technologists).

27. Why is the MLO preferred to the ML as a routine projection?

(A) The MLO visualizes the medial breast.

(B) The ML does not visualize the medial breast.

(C) The ML poorly visualizes the posterior and lateral breast.

(D) The MLO does not distort the anterior structure of the breast.

28. Which projection best shows the extreme medial aspect of the breast?

(A) CC

(B) MLO

(C) ML

(D) CV

29. In which modified projection is the superior aspect of the breast rolled medially?

(A) RM

(B) RL

(C) M

(D) LM

30. In the LMO projection the beam is directed from the

(A) upper inner aspect to the lower outer aspect of the breast

(B) inner outer aspect to the upper outer aspect of the breast

(C) lower outer aspect to the upper inner aspect of the breast

(D) superiolateral aspect to the inferomedial aspect of the breast

31. Identify the projection shown in Figure 5–6.

(A) MLO

(B) CV

(C) LM

(D) ML

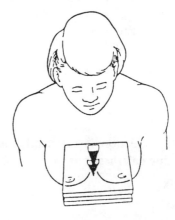

Figure 5–6. (© 2000 The American Registry of Radiologic Technologists.)

32. Identify the projection shown in Figure 5–7.

(A) RM

(B) CV

(C) RL

(D) MLO

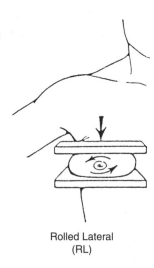

Rolled Lateral
(RL)

Figure 5–7.   (© 2000 The American Registry of Radiologic Technologists.)

33. Which projection is especially useful when analyzing calcifications?

(A) RM

(B) M

(C) LM

(D) ML

34. Identify the projection shown in Figure 5–8.

(A) RM

(B) CV

(C) RL

(D) MLO

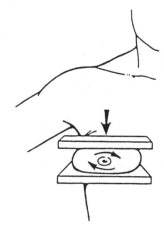

Figure 5–8.   (© 2000 The American Registry of Radiologic Technologists.)

35. All of the following statements about magnification are true EXCEPT

(A) With magnification, patient dose increases.

(B) Magnification can be used to image specimen radiographs.

(C) Magnification can be used to assess suspicious lesions.

(D) Magnification images the entire breast with one exposure.

36. In the RS position the _____ surface of the breast is rolled _____.

(A) bottom/superiorly

(B) top/inferiorly

(C) bottom/inferiorly

(D) top/inferiorly

37. Which technique accurately describes how the breast is rolled for the RM?

(A) The top is rolled medially and the bottom does not move.

(B) The top is rolled laterally and the bottom is rolled medially.

(C) The bottom is rolled medially and the top does not move.

(D) The bottom is rolled laterally and the top is rolled medially.

38. A patient with pectus excavatum may present a positioning problem because the patient has

    (A) extensive pectoral muscle
    (B) barrel chest
    (C) depressed pectoral muscle
    (D) depressed chest

39. In imaging the augmented breast in the CC position, using the modified implant-displaced technique, the breast tissue is pushed

    (A) anteriorly
    (B) posteriorly
    (C) inferiorly
    (D) superiorly

40. A routine series on patients with encapsulated implants could include an additional projection such as the

    (A) AT
    (B) CC
    (C) MLO
    (D) ML

41. Which technique is used to spread out the tissue and improve resolution on a localized area of interest?

    (A) CV
    (B) AT
    (C) TAN
    (D) spot compression

42. How many projections are routinely required to image a patient with augmented breasts?

    (A) 5
    (B) 6
    (C) 7
    (D) 8

43. When is imaging of the irradiated breast recommended?

    (A) immediately after treatment
    (B) 1–2 months after treatment
    (C) 6–12 months after treatment
    (D) 1–2 years after treatment

44. Which technique can be used with any projection with or without magnification?

    (A) spot compression
    (B) XCCL
    (C) AT
    (D) CV

45. In addition to the routine series, most post-mastectomy patients will also need a

    (A) CC
    (B) MLO
    (C) ML
    (D) CV

46. The standard projection taken on patients with breast implants requires compression

    1. for immobilization only
    2. to separate the breast tissue
    3. to assess areas of lumps

    (A) 1 only
    (B) 2 only
    (C) 1 and 3 only
    (D) 2 and 3 only

47. The specimen is radiographed to

    (A) confirm that the lesion was removed
    (B) compare various needle localization techniques
    (C) magnify the lesion to assess any possible microcalcifications
    (D) check the position of the lesion

48. The specimen is compressed to

    (A) reduce motion unsharpness
    (B) reduce radiation exposure
    (C) reduce tissue thickness
    (D) reduce magnification

49. Which procedure is performed to obtain cellular material from a suspicious area for cytologic analysis?

    (A) Ductography
    (B) Needle localization
    (C) Pneumocystogram
    (D) Fine needle aspiration

50. Preoperative localization will

    1. direct the surgeon to the area requiring biopsy
    2. help the surgeon to excise a smaller specimen
    3. verify that the correct area will be removed

       (A) 1 and 2 only
       (B) 2 and 3 only
       (C) 1 and 3 only
       (D) 1, 2, and 3

51. Core biopsy techniques developed as an alternative to surgical biopsy because this technique provided a larger sample of the area of suspicion and thus more information than

    (A) ductography
    (B) needle localization
    (C) pneumocystogram
    (D) fine needle aspiration

52. An ultrasound of a lesion showed a spherical mass with smooth regular borders, anechoic interior, and acoustic enhancement. The lesion is likely to be a

    (A) fibroadenoma
    (B) abscess
    (C) cyst
    (D) ductal carcinoma

53. In ultrasound the term *acoustic enhancement* refers to

    (A) a structure without internal echoes
    (B) a structure with internal echoes
    (C) the amount of sound passing through a structure
    (D) few echoes within a structure

54. A procedure whereby the lactiferous duct is cannulated and a small amount of contrast is injected into the duct is termed

    (A) ductography
    (B) needle localization
    (C) pneumocystogram
    (D) fine needle aspiration

55. A patient had an ultrasound, which confirmed the presence of a cyst in the breast. The radiologist wished to rule out intracystic tumor. What additional study is likely to be recommended?

    (A) Ductography
    (B) Needle localization
    (C) Pneumocystogram
    (D) Fine needle aspiration

Answers and Explanations

1. **(A)** CC projection determines whether the lesion is medial or lateral and how far it is from the nipple. The MLO or ML determines if the abnormality is superior or inferior to the nipple and how far posterior it is. The TAN projection skims the area of interest and is best used to determine if a suspected abnormality is located in the breast or the skin of the breast. *(ACR, pp. 43–49; Andolina, pp. 233, 271)*

2. **(A)** The MLO best demonstrates the posterior and upper-outer quadrants of the breast. However, it may not be possible to image the medial area on all patients in the MLO projection. The CC projection will cover this portion of medial tissue that is most likely to be missed on the MLO. *(ACR, p. 43; Andolina, pp. 198–205)*

3. **(C)** The PNL measures the perpendicular distance from the nipple to the visualized pectoral muscle on the MLO or to the edge of the film on the CC (Figure 5–9). This measurement on the MLO should be within 1 cm of the measurement on the CC projection. *(ACR , pp. 43–49; Andolina, p. 178)*

4. **(D)** In general, guidelines for the MLO include all of the statements. Additionally, the breast should not droop on the image. It may not be possible to meet all these guidelines on all patients. If one or more of these guideline elements are missing, the mammographer or radiologist must determine whether a third projection is necessary. *(ACR, pp. 34–42; Andolina, p. 202)*

5. **(B)** If the C-arm is raised too high the patient will be unable to lean forward and relax. This

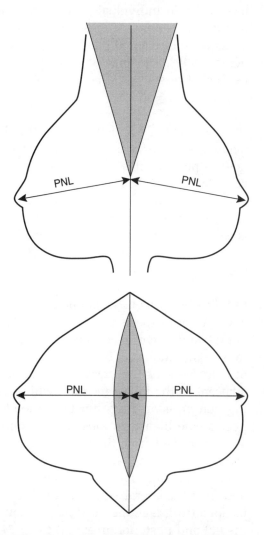

Figure 5–9. Showing the PNL. Measurement of the PNL on the MLO projection should be within 1 cm of the PNL measurement on the CC projection.

results in loss of the posterior and inferior breast tissue. If the C-arm is too low the breast droops and superior and posterior tissue is lost. *(Andolina, p. 187)*

6. **(B)** The MLO best visualizes the posterior and upper-outer quadrants of the breast while allowing distortion and overlap of the anterior structures. However, it is the best projection to visualize the maximum amount of breast tissue in a single view. *(ACR, p. 34; Andolina, p. 198)*

7. **(D)** In imaging the MLO the edge of the image recorder is placed parallel to the oblique line formed by pectoral muscle. This oblique line varies in individuals; tall, thin patients require steeper angulations (60–70°), average patients require 40–50°, and short, heavy patients 30–40°. The angle is usually the same for both breasts. *(ACR, pp. 60–62; Andolina, p. 198)*

8. **(B)** The MLO or ML determines if the abnormality is superior or inferior to the nipple and how far posterior it is. The CC or XCCL projections determine whether the lesion is medial or lateral and how far it is from the nipple. The TAN projection skims the area of interest and is best used to determine if a suspected abnormality is located in the breast or the skin of the breast. *(ACR, pp. 43–49; Andolina, p. 233, 271)*

9. **(A)** The breast is least mobile at the medial and superior aspects and most mobile at the lateral and inferior aspects. To image the maximum amount of breast tissue, the most mobile parts of the breast must be placed adjacent to the image recorder while applying compression from the least mobile aspect of the breast. In most cases, compression is applied from the superior aspect for the CC projections—(to image the maximum amount of superior and posterior breast) and from the lateral aspect for the MLO projections (to image the maximum amount of medial and posterior breast). *(ACR, p. 34; Andolina, pp. 187, 200)*

10. **(A)** The C-arm of the image receptor must be placed at the level of the elevated inframammary fold or crease. If the C-arm is raised too high, the patient will be unable to lean forward and relax. This results in loss of posterior and inferior breast tissue. If the C-arm is

too low, the breast droops and superior and posterior tissue are lost. *(Andolina, p. 187)*

11. **(D)** In imaging for the MLO, the edge of the image recorder is placed parallel to the oblique line formed by pectoral muscle. This oblique line varies in individuals; tall, thin patients require steeper angulations (60–70°), average patients require 40–50° degrees, and short, heavy patients 30–40°. The angle is usually the same for both breasts. *(ACR, pp. 60–62; Andolina, p. 198)*

12. **(A)** In the CC projection the beam is directed superiorly to inferiorly, without angulation. *(Andolina, p. 187; ACR, pp. 43–49)*

13. **(B)** Having the patient hold the supporting bars stabilizes the patient and helps to bring medial breast tissue closer to the image receptor. This is important because eliminating medial breast tissue from the CC projection may eliminate this tissue from the study. *(Wentz, pp. 58–60; Andolina, p. 188)*

14. **(A)** The RLMO is a useful alternative to the RMLO in patient with prior pacemaker surgery, open-heart surgery, or any other painful scarring along the sternum where the compression paddle would cause discomfort. The LMO projection is a reverse of the MLO and gives the same view of the anatomical structures. *(Andolina, p. 217)*

15. **(D)** The AT or axilla projection demonstrates the axillary contents or tail of the breast. This projection is especially useful in demonstrating swollen lymph nodes (lymphadenopathy). The study may be unilateral or bilateral. *(Andolina, p. 230; Wentz, p. 66)*

16. **(B)** The TAN projection is used to skim the area of interest. The projection demonstrates skin calcifications or any area free of superimposition. The TAN projection also brings the area closer to the image receptor. Before obtaining a TAN projection, the abnormality must be palpable or visualized on another projection to determine its approximate location. *(Andolina, p. 33)*

17. **(A)** With the nipple in profile, both the ML and the LM projections give a true representation of breast structures in relation to the nipple. The LM projection is best suited to image medially located abnormalities; the ML images lateral abnormalities best. In addition, unlike the image produced with the ML, the resultant image from the LM is similar to the MLO. *(Andolina, p. 225; Wentz, p. 64)*

18. **(B)** The XCCL will best image the posterolateral tissue of the breast, which may not be visualized on the CC. *(Andolina, p. 191; Wentz, p. 65)*

19. **(C)** A patient with kyphosis may also have pectus excavatum (sunken chest) or barrel-chest (pigeon breast). With these patients it is rarely possible to image the entire breast with the standard two views. An FB projection in such a situation is often useful. For the FB the entire mammography unit is rotated 180° and the image receptor is placed at the superior aspect of the breast. If the FB is not possible because of limitations of the mammography unit, the CC should be performed to image as much medial tissue as possible in addition to the MLO and LMO or LM for lateral tissue. *(Andolina, p. 251)*

20. **(B)** When comparing the MLO to the ML in search for an abnormality, medial lesions move up on the lateral from their position on the MLO; lateral lesions move down on the lateral from their position on the MLO. Centrally located lesions show little or no movement. *(Andolina, p. 265)*

21. **(D)** Milk of calcium deposits are benign calcifications that occur in microcysts as radiopaque particles mixed with fluid. On the CC projection, they appear as ill-defined calcifications. On true lateral projections, the radiopaque particles settle to the dependent portion of the cyst forming crescent- or teacup-shaped calcifications. These may be clustered, scattered, or occur bilaterally. *(Andolina, p. 171)*

22. **(B)** The TAN projection is used to skim the area of interest. The projection demonstrates skin calcification or any area free of superimposition. The TAN projection also brings the area closer to the image receptor. *(Andolina, p. 33; Wentz, p. 70)*

23. **(D)** The AT projection is an anterior-posterior projection used to visualize the axillary area or tail of the breast. Generally, steep angulation (70–90°), depending on the patient's body, is used. *(Andolina, p. 230; Wentz, p. 66)*

24. **(B)** The XCCL can be used to image the extreme posterolateral tissue missed on the CC. As with the CC projection, the beam is directed superiorly to inferiorly. *(Andolina, p. 191; Wentz, pp. 65–66)*

25. **(A)** The caudal-cranial (FB) projection is the opposite of the CC and can be used to image nonconforming patients, such as those with extreme kyphosis. The FB also places lesions high on the chest wall closer to the image receptor, providing more detail of the lesion. Patients with implants require the implant-displaced projections. *(Andolina, p. 194; Wentz, pp. 64–65)*

26. **(C)** The LM projection gives a true representation of breast structure in relation to the nipple. The LM places medially located lesions close to the image recorder. For the LM the beam is directed laterally to medially. *(Andolina, p. 25)*

27. **(C)** The MLO projection gives a distorted and overlapping view of the anterior structures of the breast, but it is the single best projection used to image the breast in its entirety. The MLO is also best at visualizing the posterior and upper-outer quadrants of the breast. The ML is poor at visualizing the most posterior and lateral parts of the breast and is not useful in visualizing areas of the breast missed on the MLO. *(Andolina, pp. 198, 219)*

28. **(D)** The CV projection is the best at imaging the extreme medial aspect of the breast. *(Andolina, p. 233; Wentz, pp. 65–66)*

29. **(A)** The rolled views help to move superimposed breast tissue away from a suspected lesion. The breast is rolled in equal and opposite directions through physical manipulation of the patient's breast. The rolled projections can be performed in any direction. For the RM, the upper surface of the breast is rolled medially and the lower surface is rolled laterally. For the RL the upper surface is rolled laterally and the lower surface is rolled medially. *(Andolina, p. 243; Wentz, pp. 68–69)*

30. **(C)** The LMO is a reverse of the MLO and results in a similar image. For the LMO, the beam is directed from the inferolateral (lower outer) aspect of the breast to the superomedial (upper inner) aspect. *(ACR, p. 71; Andolina, p. 217)*

31. **(B)** The CV is a cranial-caudal projection used to image the extreme medial aspect of the breast.

32. **(C)** In the rolled views, the breast is rolled in equal and opposite directions via physical manipulation of the patient's breast. For the RM, the upper surface of the breast is rolled medially and the lower surface is rolled laterally. For the RL, the upper surface is rolled laterally and the lower surface is rolled medially. *(Andolina, p. 243; Wentz, pp. 68–69)*

33. **(B)** Magnification mammography (M) is especially useful in assessing or finding breast calcifications, or to better outline the borders of masses. *(Andolina, p. 185)*

34. **(A)** In the rolled projections, the breast is rolled in equal and opposite directions via physical manipulation of the patient's breast. For the RM, the upper surface of the breast is rolled medially and the lower surface is rolled laterally. For the RL, the upper surface is rolled laterally and the lower surface is rolled medially. *(Andolina, p. 243; Wentz, pp. 68–69)*

35. **(D)** With magnification, the breast may be magnified up to twice its original size; therefore, the entire breast is rarely imaged. The

patient dose increases because the breast is closer to the source and additional exposure is required because of reciprocity law failure. Magnification can be used to image specimens and lesions to assess the borders or the presence of calcifications. *(Andolina, p. 185; Carlton, p. 582)*

36. **(C)** For the RS, the upper surface is rolled superiorly and the lower surface is rolled inferiorly. For the RI, the upper surface of the breast is rolled inferiorly and the lower surface is rolled superiorly. *(Andolina, p. 243; Wentz, pp. 68–69)*

37. **(D)** For the RM, the upper surface of the breast is rolled medially and the lower surface is rolled laterally. For the RL, the upper surface is rolled laterally and the lower surface is rolled medially. *(Andolina, p. 243; Wentz, pp. 68–69)*

38. **(D)** A patient with pectus excavatum has a sunken sternum and rib cage, which make imaging the medial breast tissue difficult. *(Andolina, p. 251)*

39. **(B)** In the modified implant-displaced (ID) projections, the prosthesis is displaced posteriorly and superiorly against the chest wall while gently pulling the breast tissue anterior to the prosthesis, onto the image receptor, and holding it in place with the compression device. *(ACR, p. 73; Andolina, p. 228)*

40. **(D)** The routine series for an implant patient includes the routine CC, routine MLO, CC with ID, and MLO with ID. It may be difficult to displace the implant on some patients, especially if the implant is encapsulated. If it cannot be adequately displaced, another projection (such as the 90° lateral with the implant included) should be added to the routine CC and MLO implant-included views. Imaging the patient in three projections ensures visualization of some parts of all four quadrants of the breast. The AT could be used to evaluate silicone spread into the lymph nodes; the MLO and CC are routine views. *(ACR, p. 73; Andolina, p. 220)*

41. (D) The spot compression projection focuses the compression on a single area to improve resolution and evenly spread out the breast tissues. This is sometimes useful in eliminating pseudomasses. *(ACR, p. 54; Wentz, p. 71)*

42. (D) The routine series for an implant patient includes the routine CC, routine MLO, CC with ID, and MLO with ID. The total projections per patient would therefore be eight. *(ACR, p. 73; Andolina, p. 220)*

43. (C) Radiation-induced changes in the breast usually peak at 6 months after treatment, but may continue for up to 1 year. Initially, the breast may exhibit erythema and edema, or it may harden. The breast may also be extremely sensitive and distorted because of surgery. Although the mammography examination must be adapted for each patient, a mammogram is not recommended earlier than 6 months after radiation treatment. *(Andolina, p. 260)*

44. (A) The spot compression projection focuses compression on a single area to improve resolution and evenly spread out the breast tissues. This is sometimes useful in eliminating pseudomasses. Spot compression can be taken with or without magnification and in any projection. *(ACR, p. 54; Wentz, p. 71)*

45. (C) With postmastectomy imaging, it is no longer possible to make a comparison between two "mirror-image" breasts. Therefore, an additional projection will give the radiologist a better opportunity to diagnose cancer. The ML or LM is often the preferred additional projection. *(Andolina, p. 260)*

46. (A) Caution should be used when compressing implants to avoid implant rupture. Compression should therefore be used for immobilization only and not to separate breast tissue structures. Tangential projections and magnification could be used to evaluate lumps and calcifications, respectively. The modified compression technique is used to image portions of the breast that would not be visualized because of superimposition of the implant (Figure 5–10). *(Andolina, p. 305)*

47. (A) The specimen is radiographed to ensure that the lesion was removed. The lesion should be circled on the radiograph and all the borders checked to confirm that the entire lesion was removed. *(Andolina, p. 320)*

48. (C) Compression of the specimen reduces tissue thickness, thus improving contrast. Structures are spread out, and tissue density is uniform with less superimposition of structures. The specimen can also be magnified to view calcifications. The overall effect is improved visualization and a more uniform density. *(Andolina, p. 319)*

49. (D) Fine needle aspiration (FNA) obtains cellular material for cytologic analysis. FNA uses small-gauge needles (23-gauge), which limit the amount of cells that can be aspirated. The accuracy of the procedure depends on the radiologist performing the examination and the cytologist interpreting the results. *(Andolina, p. 332; Wentz, p. 87)*

50. (D) Preoperative localization is performed on nonpalpable lesions or suspicious areas that are identified only mammographically. The radiologist assists the surgeon by placing a wire in the suspected tissue as a guide for the surgeon. The surgeon is then able to excise only the lesion and surrounding margins rather than a larger area of the breast. Once excised, the wire in the area of suspicion confirms that the correct area was removed. *(Andolina, p. 314)*

51. (D) Core biopsy provides a larger sample of breast tissue for histologic study. The larger sample (generally an 11- to 14-gauge needle is used) offers a more definitive diagnosis when compared with FNA. *(Andolina, p. 332)*

52. (C) A fibroadenoma usually has low-level internal echoes and the borders may be smooth, round, or lobulated. An abscess will be fluid filled and usually has some internal echoes. Their borders are generally well-defined, but irregular. Ductal carcinomas typically are taller than they are wide—benign masses spread out horizontally. Cancers have a spicu-

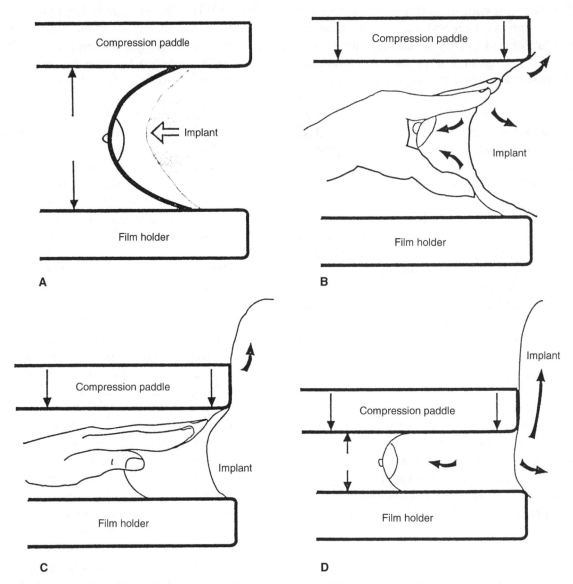

Figure 5–10. Diagram of the Eklund method. The modified compression or Eklund method for implants displaces the implant posteriorly and superiorly to image the breast tissue free of the implant. (A) Normal compression. (B and C) Displacing the implant posteriorly and superiorly prior to compression. (D) Compression of the breast tissue free of implant.

lated outline with alternating echopenic and echogenic straight lines radiating from the surface of the mass (*echopenic* means there are few echoes within a structure; *echogenic* describes a structure that produces echoes; *anechoic* means no internal echoes). A cyst has smooth walls that are enhanced through transmission. Sound traveling through a fluid-filled structure is barely attenuated; the structures distal to a cystic lesion appear to have more echoes that neighboring areas. This process is also referred to as *distal echo enhancement*. It is rare for calcifications in a cyst wall or debris within the cyst to present through transmission. *(Sanders, p. 417)*

53. **(C)** If the sound traveling through a cyst is barely attenuated, then the structure distal to the cyst appears to have more echoes than neighboring areas. The phenomenon is referred to as *acoustic enhancement* or *through transmission. (Sanders, p. 417)*

54. **(A)** Ductography or galactography is conducted on patients with nipple discharge. A small amount of contrast is injected into the duct and radiographs are taken in the craniocaudal and lateral positions. The contrast outlines these structures to visualize any pathology. *(Andolina, p. 324; Wentz, p. 86)*

55. **(C)** A pneumocystogram may be performed in conjunction with cyst aspiration. Air is injected into the cyst, which has been emptied. The inner walls of the cyst can then be assessed. In general, the air is reabsorbed by the body within a week. Ductography examines the ducts; needle localization and fine needle aspiration are used to locate nonpalpable lesions. *(Andolina, p. 324; Tabár, p. 89)*

CHAPTER 6

Practice Test 1
Questions

1. A CBE and BSE are similar in that both

    (A) involve looking and feeling for changes in the breast
    (B) are done by a trained medical professional
    (C) are done monthly
    (D) are done yearly

2. The most common cause of undercompression is

    (A) a faulty compression paddle
    (B) inadequate compression by the technologist
    (C) patient pain tolerance level
    (D) broken automatic compression device

3. In establishing processor quality control, the high average density is generally the density closest to

    (A) but not less than 2.20
    (B) but not less than 1.20
    (C) but not less than 0.45
    (D) 2.20

4. Ductal papilloma is

    (A) a benign proliferation of tissue in the male breast
    (B) a malignant tumor involving the ducts
    (C) a collection of blood in the breast, which can occur after surgery
    (D) benign growths involving the milk ducts

5. The large air gap used in magnification functions to

    1. reduce scatter
    2. improve contrast
    3. increase scatter

    (A) 1 and 2 only
    (B) 1 and 3 only
    (C) 2 and 3 only
    (D) 1, 2, and 3

6. In high-contrast imaging,

    (A) skin detail is easily seen
    (B) bright light is needed to see skin detail
    (C) glandular tissue and skin detail are seen equally
    (D) glandular tissue and skin detail are seen poorly

7. Which of the following techniques could be used to image extremely small breasts in the CC position?

    (A) Spatula
    (B) Coat hanger
    (C) Cleavage
    (D) XCCL

8. In the TAN projection the degree of obliquity depends on

    (A) the size of the patient's breast
    (B) the location of the abnormality
    (C) the location of the nipple in relation to the abnormality
    (D) whether the abnormality is palpable or nonpalpable

9. The most common physical symptom of breast cancer is

   (A) skin irritation
   (B) inverted nipples
   (C) a painless mass
   (D) a painful mass

10. Mammography is more accurate in

    (A) premenopausal women
    (B) postmenopausal women
    (C) women with fibrocystic breast
    (D) women with dense breast tissue

11. In taking medical history, hormones (both natural and artificial) are taken into account because

    1. hormones cause breast cancer
    2. early menarche increases the risk of breast cancer
    3. contraceptive use can increase breast cancer risk

       (A) 1 and 2 only
       (B) 2 and 3 only
       (C) 1 and 3 only
       (D) 1, 2, and 3

12. One major difference between the collimation in mammography and the collimation in general radiography is that

    (A) in mammography the entire image receptor area is exposed
    (B) decreasing collimation increases exposure in mammography
    (C) mammography uses a variety of beam-limiting devices
    (D) in radiography the image receptor determines field size

13. Two film emulsions are compared on a characteristic curve. The higher contrast film will

    (A) have the steeper slope
    (B) have a longer toe
    (C) shift to the right of the lower contrast film
    (D) shift to the left of the lower contrast film

14. When cleaning the intensifying screens the loaded cassette is unloaded under safelight conditions in the darkroom. The film in the cassette is

    (A) stored in the film bin during the cleaning process
    (B) removed from the cassette and discarded
    (C) returned to the cassette after cleaning
    (D) returned to the film bin

15. The retromammary space is filled with

    (A) supportive and connecting tissue
    (B) adipose tissue
    (C) fibroglandular tissue
    (D) blood vessels

16. The fatty versus fibroglandular nature of breast tissue is affected by which of the following?

    1. Age
    2. Hormone use
    3. Number of pregnancies

       (A) 1 and 2 only
       (B) 2 and 3 only
       (C) 1 and 3 only
       (D) 1, 2, and 3

17. In compression on the XCCL projection the affected arm should

    (A) not be raised, but rest along the top of the image receptor
    (B) be raised, and rest along the top of the image receptor
    (C) be place on the patient's hips
    (D) be placed according to the wishes and comfort of the patient

18. In the CC position the pectoral muscle is seen

    (A) all the time
    (B) rarely if ever
    (C) about 20% of the time
    (D) never

19. Between ages 20 and 39, a woman should have a CBE every

    (A) year
    (B) 2 years
    (C) 3 years
    (D) 4 years

20. The lesion seen in Figure 6–1 is not palpable and is not associated with nipple or skin changes. It is likely to be

    (A) invasive ductal breast carcinoma
    (B) a mammographically malignant tumor
    (C) a mammographically benign tumor
    (D) nonspecific; further testing is indicated

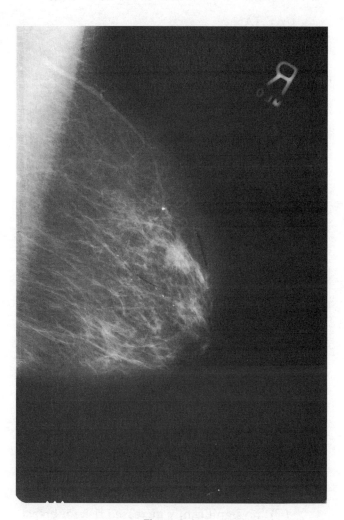

Figure 6–1.

21. Regardless of the reason, if the proper amount of compression cannot be applied

    (A) the patient must be told
    (B) the patient's doctor must be told
    (C) the radiologist must be told
    (D) it should be noted on the patient's history form

22. Magnification is contraindicated in

    1. women with thick and dense breast tissue
    2. specimen radiography
    3. normal/routine imaging

    (A) 1 and 2 only
    (B) 1 and 3 only
    (C) 2 and 3 only
    (D) 1, 2, and 3

23. If no previous mammograms are available for comparison the AEC detector should be placed

    (A) behind the nipple under a compressed area of the breast
    (B) as close to the chest wall as possible
    (C) toward the medial aspect of the breast
    (D) anywhere—placement will not affect the exposure

24. Which section of the breast is poorly visualized on the CC projection?

    (A) Lateral
    (B) Axial
    (C) Medial
    (D) Superior

25. Identify the projection in Figure 6–2.

    (A) MLO
    (B) ML
    (C) XCCL
    (D) RM

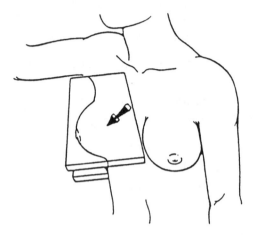

Figure 6–2. (© 2000 The American Registry of Radiologic Technologists.)

26. Generally, manual technique is sometimes necessary when imaging implants because

    (A) the implant covers the AEC detector
    (B) patients with implants have small breasts
    (C) patients with implants may have mastectomy or lumpectomy
    (D) the implant does not cover the AEC detector

27. Which projection could be used to demonstrate a deep medial lesion not seen on the CC?

    (A) AT
    (B) XCCL
    (C) CV
    (D) MLO

28. After a routine four-view mammographic series, the nipple is not seen in profile on any of the images. Additional views are done if

    1. the nipple is indistinguishable from a mass
    2. measurements for a needle localization are needed
    3. the nipple is not marked with a BB (lead shot)

       (A) 1 and 2 only
       (B) 2 and 3 only
       (C) 1 and 3 only
       (D) 1, 2, and 3

29. Identify the projection in Figure 6–3.

    (A) TAN
    (B) FB
    (C) XCCL
    (D) ML

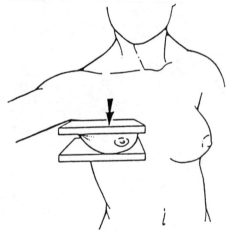

Figure 6–3. (© 2000 The American Registry of Radiologic Technologists.)

30. Your patient's sister had breast cancer. Your patient is considered to have

    (A) a greater risk for breast cancer
    (B) a minor risk for breast cancer
    (C) no significantly increased risk for breast cancer
    (D) a personal history of breast cancer

31. Per the MQSA, the average glandular dose received per view during routine screen-film mammography cannot exceed

    (A) 100 mrad
    (B) 200 mrad
    (C) 300 mrad
    (D) 400 mrad

32. When imaging an extremely dense breast using AEC, the exposure sometimes terminates, resulting in an underexposed film because of the action of the

    (A) exposure timer
    (B) backup timer
    (C) phototimer
    (D) device timer

33. The operating level density difference for the phantom should be at least

    (A) 0.40
    (B) 0.80
    (C) 0.02
    (D) 1.20

34. A film was accidentally bent prior to loading into the mammography cassette. If this film is used in mammography screening, an artifact would appear as

    (A) a minus-density artifact
    (B) a plus-density artifact
    (C) static
    (D) lines parallel to the direction of film travel

35. Montgomery glands are specialized

    (A) sweat glands
    (B) sebaceous gland
    (C) Cooper's ligaments
    (D) hair follicles

36. A woman taking estrogen replacement therapy may notice changes in the breast such as

    1. breast enlargement
    2. lumpy breast
    3. cysts

    (A) 1 and 2 only
    (B) 2 and 3 only
    (C) 1 and 3 only
    (D) 1, 2, and 3

37. Paget's disease of the breast is a (an)

    (A) infiltrating carcinoma generally limited to the breast
    (B) form of carcinoma associated with changes of the nipple
    (C) benign breast condition that is relatively common
    (D) malignant form of breast carcinoma involving the lobules

38. Variation in compression levels causes

    1. inadequate exposure on one portion of the breast
    2. over- or underexposure in other portions of the breast
    3. adequate exposure throughout the breast

    (A) 1 and 2 only
    (B) 2 and 3 only
    (C) 1 and 3 only
    (D) 1, 2, and 3 only

39. What is the major disadvantage of magnification?

    (A) reduced resolution of the image
    (B) increased patient dose
    (C) increased scattered radiation
    (D) none of the above

40. Selection of rhodium anode/filter combination for a fatty breast

    1. overpenetrates the fatty breast
    2. alters the penetrating power of the beam
    3. results in loss of contrast

       (A) 1 and 2 only
       (B) 1 and 3 only
       (C) 2 and 3 only
       (D) 1, 2, and 3

41. When taking an MLO view, drooping breast is a result of which of the following?

    1. too much compression of the anterior breast
    2. too little compression of the anterior breast
    3. compression of the posterior breast

       (A) 1 and 2 only
       (B) 2 and 3 only
       (C) 1 and 3 only
       (D) 1, 2, and 3

42. In which modified projection is the breast rolled medially?

    (A) RM
    (B) RL
    (C) M
    (D) LM

43. Factors that lower breast cancer risk include

    1. having your first childbirth at over age 30
    2. breast-feeding your child
    3. late menarche

       (A) 1 and 2 only
       (B) 2 and 3 only
       (C) 1 and 3 only
       (D) 1, 2, and 3

44. The minimum and maximum kVp of a mammography unit depends on which main factor(s)?

    (A) Radiologist preference or recommendations
    (B) Characteristics of the screen-film combination
    (C) Processing and the patient's breast size
    (D) Target and filtration material selected

45. For the daily processor quality control the mid-density should remain within

    (A) ±0.15 of the established levels
    (B) ±0.10 of the established levels
    (C) +0.30 of the established levels
    (D) +0.03 of the established levels

46. Gynecomastia defines

    (A) a localized abscess
    (B) increased breast tissue in the male breast
    (C) decreased breast tissue in the female breast
    (D) a risk of carcinoma for the male patient

47. Total filtration with a rhodium target filtration combination is

    (A) the added filtration plus the inherent filtration
    (B) equal to the added filtration
    (C) equal to the inherent filtration
    (D) the added filtration minus the inherent filtration

48. According to MQSA regulations, which of the following is not required on the final mammographic image?

    (A) Date of the examination
    (B) Technical factors used
    (C) Technologist identification
    (D) Cassette/screen identification

49. The inframammary crease is located at approximately the level of the

    (A) 2nd to 3rd rib
    (B) 3rd to 4th rib
    (C) 4th to 5th rib
    (D) 6th to 7th rib

50. Identify Cooper's ligament in Figure 6–4.

    (A) Site A
    (B) Site B
    (C) Site C
    (D) Site D

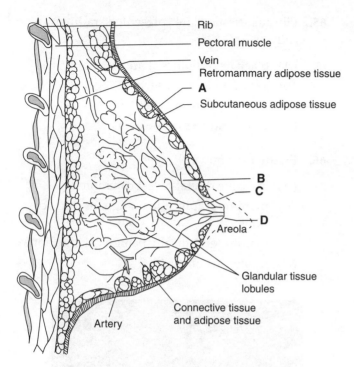

Rib
Pectoral muscle
Vein
Retromammary adipose tissue
A
Subcutaneous adipose tissue

B
C

D
Areola

Glandular tissue
lobules

Connective tissue
and adipose tissue
Artery

Figure 6–4.

51. Identify the lactiferous sinus in Figure 6–4.

(A) Site A
(B) Site B
(C) Site C
(D) Site D

52. Scattered radiation is reduced during magnification by

(A) using a small focal spot size
(B) using a grid
(C) using the air-gap technique
(D) increasing the SID

53. The purpose of ductography is to determine

1. the location of the lesions
2. if a lesion is benign or malignant
3. the number of lesions

(A) 1 only
(B) 1 and 2 only
(C) 1 and 3 only
(D) 2 and 3 only

54. In the CC projection, a technique especially useful in imaging lesions deep in the outer aspect of the breast, to include the axillary tail, on a patient whose shoulder is in the way of the compression paddle is

(A) 5° lateral tube angle
(B) 5° medial angle
(C) using a straight tube
(D) the ML projection

55. During magnification, positioning the breast away from the film utilizes which law/principle in scatter reduction?

(A) Inverse square law
(B) Reciprocity law
(C) Heel effect
(D) Line focus principle

56. A woman with one first-degree relative with breast cancer has a higher risk for breast cancer than a woman with

1. early menarche, taking oral contraceptives
2. a personal history of breast cancer
3. late menopause, on hormone replacement therapy

(A) 1 and 2 only
(B) 2 and 3 only
(C) 1 and 3 only
(D) 1, 2, and 3

57. The primary purpose of the grid in mammography is to

(A) improve image sharpness
(B) reduce the production of scatter
(C) reduce patient dose
(D) increase the contrast of the image

58. The implant-displaced (ID) projection is possible on all of the following cases EXCEPT

(A) implants placed posterior to the pectoral muscle
(B) implants placed anterior to the pectoral muscle
(C) soft implants
(D) encapsulated implants

59. A palpable mass that is not seen on a diagnostic mammogram generally means

    (A) breast cancer is ruled out; the mass is probably benign
    (B) other diagnostic testing must be considered
    (C) the mass is likely breast cancer
    (D) the mass is likely caused by fluctuating hormones

60. Which of the following patients has the greatest risk for breast cancer?

    (A) A nulliparous woman at age 40
    (B) A never-married woman
    (C) A woman, age 70
    (D) A woman, age 50 on hormone replacement therapy

61. A technologist using a 0.1-mm focal spot size is most likely performing

    (A) routine mammography work
    (B) magnification imaging
    (C) spot film imaging
    (D) stereotactic work

62. The developer temperature should always be

    (A) 95°C
    (B) 95°F
    (C) ±0.5°F (±0.3°C) of the manufacturer's recommendation
    (D) ±5.0°F (±3.0°C) of the manufacturer's recommendation

63. One box of film should be dedicated to processing quality control (QC) because

    (A) it is easier to track the repeat rate
    (B) multiple boxes introduce multiple variables
    (C) overall film density may cause fogging
    (D) films need consistent handling

64. The base of the breast refers to the

    (A) most distal point of the breast
    (B) area adjacent to the chest wall
    (C) axilla area of the breast
    (D) lower outer quadrant of the breast

65. Fibrous tissues are presented radiographically as

    (A) black or radiolucent areas
    (B) gray and less dense areas
    (C) white or denser areas
    (D) black and less dense areas

66. Figure 6–5 shows

    (A) invasive ductal breast carcinoma
    (B) mammographically malignant calcifications
    (C) mammographically benign calcifications
    (D) numerous oil cysts

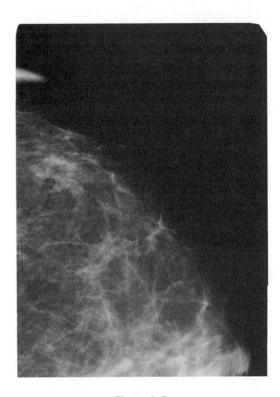

Figure 6–5.

67. The MLO projection demonstrates a large encapsulated lesion occupying almost the entire breast. The contour is sharp and the lesion is radiolucent. This lesion is most likely to be a (an)

    (A) oil cyst
    (B) hematoma
    (C) fibroadenoma
    (D) lipoma

68. In mammography the AEC detector is placed directly

    (A) above the cassette
    (B) below the grid
    (C) above the grid
    (D) below the cassette

69. Since 1989, the death rate from breast cancer has declined because

    (A) more cancers are discovered at a later stage
    (B) more cancers are discovered at an earlier stage
    (C) the long-term survival rate for breast cancer patients is stable
    (D) patients who survive 5 years will survive an additional 10

70. Contaminated developer will likely result in

    1. decreased film speed
    2. increased contrast
    3. increased film base density

        (A) 1 and 2 only
        (B) 2 and 3 only
        (C) 1 and 3 only
        (D) 1, 2, and 3

71. Spot compression

    1. applies more compression to a localized area
    2. can be performed with magnification
    3. employs a coned collimated field to limit the area of interest

        (A) 1 only
        (B) 1 and 2 only
        (C) 2 and 3 only
        (D) 1, 2, and 3

72. Identify the projection in Figure 6–6.

    (A) TAN
    (B) FB
    (C) XCCL
    (D) RM

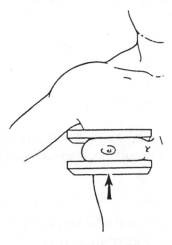

Figure 6–6. (© 2000 The American Registry of Radiologic Technologists.)

73. To reduce the possibility of imaging the abdomen in the MLO position the mammographer could

    (A) have the patient stand just at the image receptor and bend back
    (B) have the patient stand away from the image receptor and bend forward
    (C) have the patient turn medially to image the lateral breast on the CC
    (D) discard the MLO and image the breast in the lateral position instead

74. A four-view mammography series shows a solitary tumor without calcification in the UOQ of the left breast. Only the anterior margins are seen. The next step is

    (A) biopsy
    (B) spot compression
    (C) stereotactic localization
    (D) aspiration

75. Why is the specimen magnified?

    (A) To ensure that the lesion has been completely removed
    (B) To visualize the lesion within the specimen
    (C) To compare the magnified and nonmagnified views
    (D) For cytologic analysis

76. In digital mammography, an overexposed image

    (A) appears excessively noisy
    (B) is too light
    (C) is too dark
    (D) appears correctly exposed

77. Which of the following patients is likely to be diagnosed with pathologic gynecomastia?

    (A) Lactating woman
    (B) Elderly man
    (C) Premenopausal woman
    (D) Postmenopausal woman

78. Montgomery glands are located on the breast's

    (A) skin
    (B) nipple
    (C) areola
    (D) muscle

79. Extended processing increases the amount of time the film is immersed in the

    (A) developer solution
    (B) fixer solution
    (C) dryer
    (D) both the developer and fixer solutions

80. If the humidity in the dark room drops lower than 30% the result is

    (A) an increase in base fog
    (B) film scratches
    (C) static patterns on film
    (D) reduced film speed

81. Over age 40, it is recommended that women have a clinical breast examination every

    (A) year
    (B) 2 years
    (C) 3 years
    (D) 4 years

82. Fibrous and glandular tissues are more _____ than fatty tissue and result in areas of _____ optical density on the radiograph.

    (A) radiolucent/lower
    (B) radiolucent/higher
    (C) radiopaque/higher
    (D) radiopaque/lower

83. Compression

    1. increases spatial resolution
    2. decreases spatial resolution
    3. improves contrast

    (A) 2 only
    (B) 3 only
    (C) 1 and 3 only
    (D) 2 and 3 only

84. Which of the following involves the use of a thin needle to remove cell samples from a suspected cancerous lesion in the breast for cytologic analysis?

    (A) Core biopsy
    (B) Excisional biopsy
    (C) Needle localization
    (D) FNA

85. A lesion is superimposed by breast tissue in the CC projection. A projection used to demonstrate the lesion in the same projection free of superimposition is the

    (A) MLO
    (B) ID
    (C) XCCL
    (D) RM

86. In imaging the breast in the MLO projection, compression to the lower portion of the breast is compromised if

    1. the image receptor is too high
    2. the patient has a protruding abdomen
    3. too much axilla and shoulder are under compression

    (A) 1 and 2 only
    (B) 1 and 3 only
    (C) 2 and 3 only
    (D) 1, 2, and 3

87. Involution of the breast describes a process by which

    (A) milk is removed from the breast by suckling
    (B) breast epithelium proliferates during menstruation
    (C) breast epithelium decreases due to postmenopausal changes
    (D) estrogen causes an overall density decrease in the breast

88. Which is not a recommended method of BSE?

    (A) Wedge
    (B) Circular
    (C) Perpendicular (up and down)
    (D) Horizontal (across)

89. In the dedicated mammography unit, the single intensifying screen is positioned in contact with the film emulsion on

    (A) the side of the cassette away from the x-ray source
    (B) the side of the film facing the x-ray source
    (C) the side of the cassette facing the x-ray source
    (D) either side—the placement does not matter

90. Grid use in magnification mammography is contraindicated because

    1. grid use increases contrast
    2. scatter is already minimized
    3. the grid results in increased patient dose

    (A) 1 and 2 only
    (B) 2 and 3 only
    (C) 1 and 3 only
    (D) 1, 2, and 3

91. The breast can be imaged in the FB projection

    1. to improve visualization of lesions in uppermost aspect of breast by reducing OID
    2. during needle localization to provide shorter route to inferior lesions
    3. to maximize the amount of tissue visualized in patients with kyphosis

    (A) 1 and 2 only
    (B) 2 and 3 only
    (C) 1 and 3 only
    (D) 1, 2, and 3

92. Identify the projection in Figure 6–7.

    (A) TAN
    (B) FB
    (C) XCCL
    (D) ML

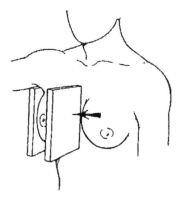

Figure 6–7. (© 2000 The American Registry of Radiologic Technologists.)

93. If the radiologist requested the nipple be imaged in profile and after a four-view series the nipple is not in profile on any of the images, the next step is to

    (A) discard the first set of mammograms and repeat the series making sure to position the nipple in profile
    (B) include the first set of mammograms and repeat the series making sure to place BB markers on the nipple
    (C) discard the first set of mammograms and repeat the CC projections with the nipple in profile
    (D) include the first set of mammograms with a repeat series of the breast showing the nipple in profile

94. Mercury in a glass-type thermometer is not recommended for use in QC testing because

    1. mercury is potentially inaccurate
    2. mercury is a potential source of contamination
    3. glass-type thermometers may break

    (A) 1 and 2 only
    (B) 2 and 3 only
    (C) 1 and 3 only
    (D) 1, 2, and 3

95. What factors are used to maintain a sharp image during magnification?

    1. Adjustable focal spot sizes
    2. Decreasing the thickness of the body part
    3. Decreasing the resolution

    (A) 1 and 2 only
    (B) 1 and 3 only
    (C) 2 and 3 only
    (D) 1, 2, and 3

96. The half-value layer (HVL) of the x-ray beam is measured with a

    (A) quality-control dosimeter
    (B) slit camera
    (C) pinhole camera
    (D) star pattern

97. The repeat rate should be analyzed if the rate changes from the previous measure rate by more than

    (A) ±2%
    (B) ±3%
    (C) ±4%
    (D) ±5%

98. A magnification view of breast shows several oval-shaped radiolucent lesions with egg-shell-like calcifications. These are most likely to be

    (A) ductal papilloma
    (B) fibroadenomas
    (C) oil cysts
    (D) hematomas

99. The image viewing environment

    1. has no effect on the detection of cancerous lesions
    2. obliterates the advantages of optimum image quality
    3. eliminates extraneous viewbox light

       (A) 1 and 2 only
       (B) 1 and 3 only
       (C) 2 and 3 only
       (D) 1, 2, and 3

100. In general, ID series are taken in

    (A) AT and MLO projections
    (B) CC and ML projections
    (C) CC and MLO projections
    (D) CC and LM projections

101. Today all technologists performing mammograms independently must have

    1. satisfied the interim requirements of the FDA
    2. completed at least 40 contact hours of documented training in mammography
    3. performed at least 25 examinations under direct supervision of a qualified technologist

       (A) 1 and 2 only
       (B) 2 and 3 only
       (C) 1 and 3 only
       (D) 1, 2, and 3

101. The criteria for a properly positioned MLO includes

    1. a concave pectoral muscle on the anterior border
    2. fat visualized posterior to the fibroglandular tissues
    3. an open inframammary fold

       (A) 1 and 2 only
       (B) 2 and 3 only
       (C) 1 and 3 only
       (D) 1, 2, and 3

103. A benign inflammatory condition of the lactiferous ducts leading to nipple discharge, nipple inversion, or periareolar sepsis is called

    (A) ductal ectasia
    (B) Paget's disease of the breast
    (C) peau d'orange
    (D) ductal papilloma

104. The cells lining the alveoli are called

    (A) epithelial cells
    (B) myoepithelial cells
    (C) basement cells
    (D) superficial cells

105. Using a cassette with poor film screen contact will result in

    (A) a noisy image
    (B) localized unsharpness
    (C) motion unsharpness
    (D) a lower contrast image

106. A technique describing reshaping of the breast is called

    (A) reduction mammoplasty
    (B) mammoplasty
    (C) breast augmentation
    (D) breast biopsy

107. A major cause of radiographic noise is

    (A) film graininess
    (B) quantum mottle
    (C) poor resolution
    (D) motion

108. Failure of the hyporetention test will result in what type of long-term artifact marks on the film?

    (A) Streaks of increased optical density
    (B) Areas of reduced density
    (C) Yellow brown stains
    (D) Round spots of increased density

109. In positioning for the SIO the _____ of the breast will rest on the image receptor.

    (A) lateral surface
    (B) base
    (C) medial surface
    (D) apex

110. Imaging males will present the same difficulty as imaging small, firm-breasted females. An added problem may be that

    (A) males have more problems with the compression
    (B) the male breast is smaller than the smallest female breast
    (C) males have more muscular breast tissue
    (D) hair on the chest of males makes compression difficult

111. For the SIO projection the central ray is directed

    (A) inferolateral to superomedial
    (B) superomedial to inferolateral
    (C) inferomedial to superolateral
    (D) superiolateral to inferomedial

112. Which of the following are considered agencies granting accreditation under the FDA regulation?

    1. ACR
    2. ARRT
    3. State accreditation bodies

    (A) 1 and 2 only
    (B) 1 and 3 only
    (C) 2 and 3 only
    (D) 1, 2, and 3

113. Which alternative projection could be used in imaging a patient with a prominent pacemaker?

    (A) ML
    (B) LMO
    (C) XCCL
    (D) MLO

114. During needle localization, breast positioning should provide the shortest skin-to-abnormality distance in order to

    1. minimize trauma to the breast
    2. ensure minimal excursion of the biopsy needle into the breast
    3. reduce the possibility of needle deflection

    (A) 1 and 2 only
    (B) 1 and 3 only
    (C) 2 and 3 only
    (D) 1, 2, and 3

115. In addition to the patient's name, all mammographic reports should have the

    1. final assessment of findings
    2. hospital number or additional patient identifier
    3. name of the radiologist

    (A) 1 and 2 only
    (B) 1 and 3 only
    (C) 2 and 3 only
    (D) 1, 2, and 3

Answers and Explanations

1. **(A)** Both the CBE and the BSE are examinations of the breast where changes in the shape, contour, and texture of the breast are assessed and the breast is checked for lumps. The CBE is done by a health professional, whereas the BSE is done by the woman on herself. The BSE should always be done monthly after age 20. The CBE is recommended every 3 years for those under 40 and every year for those over 40. *(ACR, p. 10)*

2. **(B)** Studies have shown that although there are many reasons for undercompression, the main reason is due to a lack of communication between the technologist and the patient. The technologist undercompresses the breast either because the patient refuses further compression, is unable to tolerate more compression, or the technologist wants to "protect" the patient from further pain. Patients generally tolerate more compression if they fully understand the reason for the compression. *(ACR, p. 90; Andolina, p. 34)*

3. **(A)** In calculating the density difference two average densities are used. The high average density is the density closest to, but not more than, 2.20. The low average density is the density closest to but not less than 0.45. The difference between these two densities is the density difference (DD). *(ACR, p. 151)*

4. **(D)** A papilloma generally occurs near the nipple but can occur deep within the breast. The papilloma may produce spontaneous discharge from the nipple or if deep within the breast may appear radiographically as a mass. Ductal papillomas are benign and are only visualized with ductography. *(Andolina, p. 158; Breast Cancer Resource Center: Benign Breast Conditions, p. 9)*

5. **(A)** The large air gap acts like a grid and reduces scatter, thus improving contrast. Positioning the breast away from the film takes advantage of the inverse-square law: the intensity of the scattered radiation is reduced because the distance between the film and the object is increased. *(ACR, pp. 59–60; Andolina, p. 63)*

6. **(B)** To visualize minimal changes in glandular structures, high-contrast mammography provides detail of glandular tissue, but does not show skin detail. The skin is only seen under "bright light." If the skin is seen normally, the film is underexposed, especially in the glandular regions; detail is lost and lesions may be missed. *(Andolina, p. 184)*

7. **(A)** The spatula can be used instead of the mammographer's fingers to pull extremely small breasts into position for compression. The coat hanger method can be used to pull in palpable lumps that would otherwise slip out from under the compression. Cleavage views images the extreme medial breast in the CC projection and XCCL images the extreme lateral breast in the CC projection. *(Andolina, pp. 191–194, 243)*

8. **(B)** In the TAN projection, the technique is to take a skimming projection of the area of interest. Because the TAN can be taken in any projection, the degree of obliquity and the projection depends on the location of the abnormality. The TAN can be taken in any projection (Figure 6–8). *(Andolina, p. 233)*

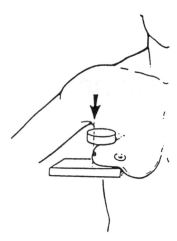

Figure 6–8. (© 2000 The American Registry of Radiologic Technologists.)

9. **(C)** Although pain can be associated with breast cancer, a painless mass is the more common symptom of breast cancer. Painful masses are associated with cysts. Less common symptoms of breast cancer include skin thickening, skin irritation or distortion, and sudden nipple inversion, discharge, erosion, or tenderness. *(ACS, p. 10)*

10. **(B)** On average a mammogram will detect 90% of breast cancers in women without symptoms and is more accurate in postmenopausal compared to premenopausal women. Some cancers are not detected mammographically because of increased breast density, as in the fibrocystic breast, faster growth rate, or failure to recognize the early signs of an abnormality. *(ACS, p. 11)*

11. **(B)** Hormone use influences breast cancer risk, but does not actually cause breast cancer. All factors that affect the reproductive hormones in a woman's body increase risk for breast cancer. *(ACS, p. 9)*

12. **(A)** In general use of any beam-limiting device in radiography or mammography requires increased exposure. Both use varying sized beam-limiting devices. However, unlike general radiography where the beam should be limited to the size of the part, in mammography the entire field (not just the breast) is exposed. This is necessary to reduce

extraneous light when viewing the image. *(Wentz, p. 22)*

13. **(A)** Characteristic curves (also called D log E, sensitometric, or Hurter and Driffield [H & D] curves) describe the relationship between the radiation exposure and the optical density produced on a film. At the toe and shoulder of the curve, large variations in exposure result in little or no change in density. In the straight-line portion of the curve (the useful region), small changes in exposure cause large changes in density. Calculations of film contrast use the average gradient or slope between two points of the curve. Films that have a steeper slope have a higher contrast. Two characteristic curves can also be used to compare film speeds (Figure 6–9). The curve that lies to the left (closer to the density axis) is faster. *(Bushong, p. 260)*

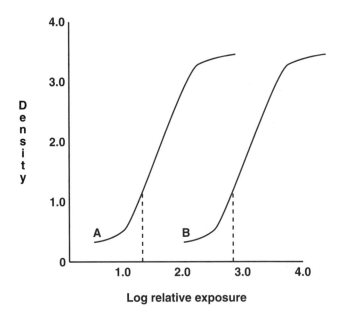

Figure 6–9. Characteristic curves. Graph of the H & D curve from two different types of radiographic films. Film A has a faster speed than film B because its speed point is the left of film B. Film B has a higher contrast than film A because the slope of its curve is steeper than that of film A.

14. **(B)** The film in the cassette should be discarded because any attached dirt from the cassette will be carried into the film bin or returned to the cassette. *(ACR, p. 149; Andolina, p. 103)*

15. **(B)** The retromammary space separates the breast from the pectoral muscle. It is filled with a layer of adipose or fatty tissue as opposed to the supporting and connective tissue (stroma), blood vessels, and various ductal structures that make up the glandular and fibrous tissues of the breast. *(Andolina, pp. 141, 150)*

16. **(D)** Generally, glandular tissues predominate in younger women and adipose or fatty tissues in older patients. This ratio is not fixed, and depends on the woman's genetic predisposition. It fluctuates with hormone levels, whether the hormonal changes are due to medication use or pregnancy, lactation, or menopause. *(Andolina, p. 143)*

17. **(A)** The purpose of the XCCL projection is to image the lateral aspect of the breast. Raising the patient's arm forces more axilla under the compression paddle. This action does not allow adequate compression of the lateral and anterior aspects of the breast. The shoulder should be relaxed and down. *(Andolina, p. 194)*

18. **(C)** Depending on patient body habitus, the pectoral muscle is imaged on the medial aspect of the breast in about 20–30% of all CC projections. It may be visualized unilateral or bilateral. Routine imaging of the pectoral muscle in the center of the breast can indicate faulty positioning with loss of medial or lateral breast tissue. *(Andolina, p. 189; Wentz, pp. 58–60)*

19. **(C)** The ACS guidelines for early detection of breast cancer includes having a clinical breast examination (CBE) every 3 years between ages 20 and 39 and every year after age 40. *(ACS, p. 11)*

20. **(D)** Whenever a large radiating structure or area of architectural distortion (even when superficial) is not associated with skin changes or nipple retraction, the mammogram is considered nonspecific, and further testing is indicated. If the lesion is palpable, malignancy cannot be ruled out. However, the lesion must be biopsied for a definitive diagnosis. This lesion is a radial scar (see Figure 6–1). Radial scars are rarely palpable and never involve skin changes. *(Tabár, p. 132)*

21. **(D)** Although the technologist should tell the radiologist, anything unusual should be charted on the patient's medical or history form. The patient's records are a means of communication between the mammographer and the radiologist and can be important legal documents used to define what was or was not done to a patient. Records can also be used as evidence in court cases. *(Wentz, p. 44)*

22. **(B)** Magnification techniques are useful in mammography to assess microcalcifications or the border of a lesion, or to image a specimen to check for calcifications. For women with thick, dense breast tissue, magnification is contraindicated because long exposure times and high kVp degrades the image. The patient also receives an unnecessarily high radiation dose. *(Andolina, p. 185; Bushong, p. 316)*

23. **(A)** If the detector is placed in a single region of adipose tissue in an otherwise glandular breast, the adipose area will be correctly exposed but the glandular area will be underexposed resulting in an increased chance of missed breast cancer. In imaging adipose and glandular tissue, the detector must be under glandular breast to obtain proper film density. Glandular tissue is distributed centrally and laterally within the breast; therefore, the AEC should be placed behind the nipple, making sure it is under an area of compressed breast. *(Andolina, pp. 143, 183; Wentz, p. 48)*

24. **(A)** All effort should be made to image the medial breast tissue on the CC mammogram; eliminating it could eliminate this area of the breast from the study. The patient should be rotated slightly medially, even if this means loosing some lateral breast tissue. Although the medial breast is imaged on the MLO, superimposition of glandular structures and increased OID often causes distortion of that area. *(Andolina, p. 198)*

25. **(A)** The MLO projection best demonstrates the posterior and upper-outer quadrants of the breast. This projection images the breast entirely, but distorts the anterior structures. *(Andolina, p. 198)*

26. **(A)** If breast tissue is over the AEC detector, automatic exposure is possible. AEC works on the principle of terminating the exposure when sufficient x-ray reaches the image receptor to produce a preset optical density. Because implants are basically radiopaque, if the implant is positioned over the AEC the tube will try to provide sufficient output to penetrate the implant and also provide optimal density. This generally leads to an excessive radiation dose to the patient. *(Bushong, p. 291)*

27. **(C)** The CV best images the medial breast. The MLO will best demonstrate the posterior and upper outer quadrant of the breast. The XCCL and AT will demonstrate the lateral and axilla portion of the breast, respectively. *(Andolina, pp. 187–230)*

28. **(A)** Putting the nipple in profile is sometimes counterproductive. Breast tissue is lost either superiorly, inferiorly, laterally, or medially, depending on the projection and the location of the nipple on the breast. Missed tissue can then lead to undetected breast cancer. If the nipple is not in profile, additional films are needed for the above reasons or if a subareolar abnormality is suspected, but should not be done solely to place the nipple in profile, even if the nipple is not marked with a BB. *(Andolina, p. 183)*

29. **(C)** The XCCL projection best images the posterolateral parts of the breast. The beam is directed superiorly to inferiorly, similar to a standard CC projection. *(Andolina, p. 191)*

30. **(A)** Although the biggest risk factor of breast cancer is gender (female) having a sister with breast cancer significantly increases risks for the disease. A personal history applies only if the patient has had breast cancer. *(ACR, pp. 8–9)*

31. **(C)** The final rules of mammography dictated by the MQSA state that a single view screen-film mammogram should not give more that 300 mrad/view average glandular dose when a grid is used and should not exceed 100 mrad/view without a grid. *(Andolina, p. 34; Bushong, p. 553)*

32. **(B)** Newer mammogram generators have a backup timer similar to the conventional AEC systems. The mammography exposure timer always attempts to get the correct density, while the phototimer (AEC) cuts the exposure when the correct density is achieved. The backup timer stops the exposure before the optimal density is reached if the energy of the beam is too low. If the backup time is reached during a breast exposure, the radiographer should select a higher kVp setting for the repeat radiograph. The primary reason the backup timer is reached is because the energy of the beam is too low to penetrate the breast. Only by selecting a higher kVp is the technologist able to increase the beam's energy. *(Carlton, p. 573)*

33. **(A)** The MQSA requires that the density difference due to the 4.0-mm acrylic disc should be at least 0.40, and should not vary by more than ±0.05 from the operating level. Also, the phantom image background optical density should be at least 1.40 and should not vary by more than ±0.20 from the operating level. *(ACR, p. 186)*

34. **(A)** White (minus-density) artifacts indicate pressure on the emulsion before exposure and dark (plus-density) artifacts indicate pressure after exposure. Static is caused by film handling in low humidity. Improperly cleaned or worn rollers causes repeating artifacts that run parallel to the direction of film travel. *(Andolina, pp. 101–103)*

35. **(A)** The Montgomery glands are seen as protrusions on the surface of the areola and are actually specialized sweat glands. They usually become more prominent during pregnancy and lactation. *(Andolina, p. 140; Harris, p. 4)*

36. **(D)** Estrogen and progesterone are two of the many hormones responsible for many physiologic changes in the breast. Estrogen is responsible for ductal proliferation and progesterone for lobular proliferation. Once a woman starts estrogen the changes can be spotty, causing lumps or increased interstitial fluids (cysts), but will generally result in an overall increase in glandular tissue. *(Andolina, p. 149)*

37. **(B)** Paget's disease of the breast (first described by Jean Paget in 1874) is a special form of ductal carcinoma associated with eczematous changes of the nipple. Generally it presents as a malignant nipple lesion. *(Tabár, p. 190)*

38. **(A)** Compression should be applied evenly over the breast by using a flat paddle parallel to the image receptor. Uneven compression leads to false-negative or false-positive results because comparison between relative mass densities is not possible. *(Andolina, p. 184)*

39. **(B)** The principle disadvantage of magnification is that the increased OID places the patient's breast very close to the x-ray tube. Because the radiation intensity is related to the square of the distance, magnification usually results in about twice the normal patient dose. The small focal spot used in magnification compensates for the reduced resolution. Magnification therefore does not decrease image resolution. The air-gap technique reduces rather than increases the amount of scattered radiation reaching the image receptor. *(Bushong, pp. 268, 304)*

40. **(D)** Mammography uses a combination of molybdenum or rhodium as target materials. Molybdenum has an atomic number of 42 versus rhodium with a slightly higher atomic number of 45. The emission spectrum from a molybdenum target tube has a slightly lower K-edge and less bremsstrahlung x-rays than that of rhodium. This difference in emission spectra allows for slightly higher kVp selections when using rhodium targets. The target material then determines the kVp range and thus the quality of the beam. Rhodium produces better images for thick, dense breast without loss of contrast and with decreased patient dose. However, if used on fatty breast the contrast will be significantly reduced with only a minimal reduction in dose. *(Andolina, p. 71; Bushong, p. 310)*

41. **(B)** The breast droops in the MLO if adequate compression is not applied to the anterior breast. Compression should be applied evenly throughout the anterior, posterior, and lateral parts of the breast. If too much axilla is included in the compression field, the posterior breast is adequately compressed, but compression is inadequate for the anterior breast. *(Andolina, p. 250; Wentz, p. 83)*

42. **(A)** In the rolled view, the top half of the breast is rolled in one direction and the bottom half in the other direction. With the medial roll, the top is rolled medially. In the lateral roll, the top is rolled laterally. The RM and RL are both useful in separating glandular structures of the breast to clear questions of superimposition. *(Andolina, p. 243)*

43. **(B)** Breast cancer risk decreases among women who have a first child prior to age 30, breast-feed, and experience late menarche or early menopause. Studies have suggested that reproductive hormones influence breast cancer; therefore, factors that affect reproductive hormones (early menarche [before 12], late menopause [over 55], late age at first full-term pregnancy [over 30], use of oral contraceptives, and estrogen replacement therapy) affect breast cancer risk. *(ACR, pp. 8–9)*

44. **(D)** All mammographic x-ray tubes are manufactured with a tungsten, molybdenum, or rhodium target. These targets have different atomic numbers and therefore different emission spectrums. The emission spectrum of the beam is shaped by altering a combination of the target material and the filtration. However, these designs are built into the mammography unit. Although the technologist can select different targets, the technologist is unable to alter the built-in target material

and therefore the emission spectrum of the beam. *(Bushong, p. 312; Wentz, p. 20)*

45. (A) The MQSA requires that the mid-density and density difference be within ±0.15 of the established operating level. The base plus fog must remain within +0.03 of the established operating level. *(ACR, p. 159)*

46. (B) Gynecomastia is a benign increase of tissue in the male breast. It can occur bilaterally or unilaterally. Gynecomastia does not increase the risk of breast cancer for male patients. *(Andolina, p. 158)*

47. (A) The total filtration is a combination of the inherent and any added filtration. In any mammography unit the inherent filtration may fall in the region of 0.1 mm Al or equivalent, but the total filtration should never be lower than 0.5 mm Al or equivalent. *(Bushong, pp. 311–312)*

48. (B) Although the MQSA recommends that technical factors appear on the film, this is not an MQSA requirement. Other recommendations are

- flash card ID versus stick-on labels because the flash ID is more permanent
- separate date stickers because they are easy to read and can be color-coded by year

The requirements are

- Name of patient and additional patient identifier
- Date of exam
- View and laterality (placed near the axilla using the standardized codes)
- Facility name and location (must include city, state, and zip code)
- Technologist identification
- Cassette/screen identification
- Mammography unit identification (if more than one unit per site) *(ACR, pp. 26–27)*

49. (D) The breast can reach superiorly from the clavicle (2nd or 3rd rib), and inferiorly to meet the abdominal wall at the level of the 6th or 7th rib. This lowest point of the breast is called the inframammary crease or fold. *(Andolina, p. 141; Harris, p. 3)*

50. (A) The Cooper's ligaments are fibrous membranes that support the lobes of the breast. The ligaments attach to the base of the breast and extend outward attaching to the anterior superficial fascia of the skin (Figure 6–10). *(Andolina, p. 140)*

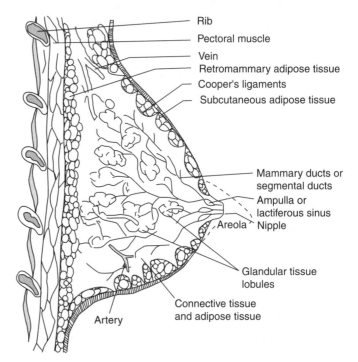

Figure 6–10.   Diagram of the breast.

51. (C) Starting at the nipple, this duct starts as a collecting duct and immediately widens into an ampulla called the lactiferous sinus. This is a pouch-like structure that again narrows and joins one or more segmental ducts, eventually branching further until it ends at the terminal ductal lobular unit. *(Andolina, p. 140)*

52. (C) Scattered radiation is produced whenever the useful beam intercepts any object causing it to diverge. There are two methods of reducing the amount of scattered radiation reaching the image recorder: limiting the x-ray field size (not an option in mammography) and the use of grids. In magnification mammography the large air gap acts as a grid in reducing scattered radiation. Grid use will therefore unnecessarily increase the exposure dose to the patient. Increasing the SID reduces magnification but does not reduce the amount of scatter production. It is not used in magnification mammography. The small focal spot is necessary to increase resolution, but this does not affect the amount of scattered radiation reaching the film. *(Bushong, pp. 221, 268)*

53. (C) Ductography will not determine if a lesion is malignant or benign but it can determine the location and number of lesions. Only a cytologic or histologic analysis can accurately determine the true nature of the lesion. *(Andolina, p. 324; Wentz, p. 86)*

54. (A) A 5° lateral tube angulation allows the compression paddle to clear the humeral head. The tube angled medially further projects the humeral head in the area of interest. Using a straight tube is a routine CC projection and does not alter the imaging. Other alternatives (XCCL) image the lateral breast or (ML) change the orientation of any abnormality in relation to the nipple. *(ACR, p. 60; Andolina, p. 194)*

55. (A) Positioning the breast away from the film takes advantage of the inverse-square law: the intensity of the scattered radiation is reduced because the distance between the film and the object is increased. The heel effect describes the process that causes the radiation intensity at the cathode side of the x-ray field to be higher than that on the anode side. The line focus principle is an angled design of the tube target that allows a large area for heating while maintaining a small focal spot. The reciprocity law states that the density produced on a radiograph is equal for any combination of mA and exposure time as long as the product of mA and the ms is equal. *(ACR, pp. 59–60; Bushong, pp. 132, 186)*

56. (C) Risk factors increase a woman's risk for breast cancer. Risk factors are divided into major and minor categories. Major risks carry a higher possibility of developing breast cancer. Major risk factors are those outside of a woman's control and include gender, age, inherited genetic risk, and family and personal history. Minor factors are those within a woman's control and include use of oral contraceptives, having a first child at over age 30, not breast-feeding, early menarche (under 12 years), or late menopause (55 or older). *(ACS, p. 8)*

57. (D) Grids do not improve image sharpness; the sharpness of an image is affected by the focal-spot size, SID, OID, type of intensifying screens, and motion. Grids increase patient dose and reduce the amount of scattered radiation striking the film, but do not affect the production of scatter radiation. Grid use will, however, increase contrast. *(Bushong, p. 315; Wentz, p. 22)*

58. (D) As long as the implant is soft and remains free of encapsulation the ID view is possible. Once the implant is encapsulated it is difficult if not impossible to displace. *(Andolina, p. 227)*

59. (B) On average a mammogram detects 90% of breast cancers in women without symptoms, and is more accurate in postmenopausal than premenopausal women. The reason some cancers are not detected mammographically include breast density, faster growth rate, or failure to recognize the early signs of an abnormality. If the mammogram is normal and the patient feels a palpable mass, the mass could be normal or abnormal. The patient must contact her doctor immediately for further testing. *(ACS, p. 11; Andolina, p. 36)*

60. (C) Risk factors increase a woman's risk for breast cancer. Risk factors are divided in major and minor categories. Major factors are those outside of a woman's control, and include gender, age, inherited genetic risk, and family and personal history. Minor factors are those within a woman's control and include not having children (nulliparity), having a first child at over age 30, not breast-feeding, early menarche (under 12 years), late menopause (55 or older), or use of hormones as birth control or therapeutically. *(ACR, pp. 8–9)*

61. **(B)** The focal spot size is important in mammography and many x-ray tubes have two focal spot sizes—one for routine and one for magnification work. In routine work, the focal spot size can be 0.4 or smaller. In magnification work, the focal spot may be 0.15 or smaller. Any work done with a 0.1-mm focal spot size would be for magnification. *(Bushong, p. 311; Wentz, p. 20)*

62. **(C)** Although the majority of processing units operate at a developer temperature of 95°F, some may not. The actual temperature is suggested by the manufacturer and should be within ±0.5°F of the value specified by the manufacturer. *(ACR, pp. 130, 215)*

63. **(B)** Daily QC is used to assess consistency of film and film processing. Introducing multiple processing variables such as variations in film emulsion (by using a film from a different box each time) will muddle the results. *(ACR, p. 149)*

64. **(B)** The breast includes the nipple, inframammary fold, and tail of Spence. The tail of Spence (tail, axilla, or axillary tail are other names used) describes the area of the breast stretching up into the axilla. The base describes the region where the inframammary fold is located, closest to the chest wall. The apex is the nipple region, and the most distal point of the breast. *(Andolina, p. 140; Harris, p. 3)*

65. **(C)** Fibrous tissue is usually described with glandular tissue together as fibroglandular densities. X-rays pass more easily through fatty tissue than through fibrous or glandular tissue. Fatty areas appear radiolucent (black or less dense area on the mammogram). The fibroglandular or fibrous tissue is more radiopaque than fatty tissue, and shows as areas

of lower optical density (white or dense) on the mammogram. *(Andolina, p. 146; Wentz, p. 12)*

66. **(B)** Figure 6–5 shows casting-type calcifications. The shape of the cast is determined by the uneven production of calcification and the irregular necrosis of the cellular debris. The contours of the cast are always irregular in density, width, and length, and the cast is always fragmented. A calcification is seen as branching when it extends into adjacent ducts. Also, the width of the ducts will determine the width of the castings. A diagnosis of invasive ductal carcinoma is only made on cytologic or histologic analysis. *(Tabár, p. 150)*

67. **(D)** The only huge radiolucent breast lesion is a lipoma. The oil cyst appears mammographically as eggshell-like calcifications. Both the fibroadenoma and the hematoma are seen as circular-oval lesions with mixed densities. *(Tabár, pp. 21, 28)*

68. **(D)** The AEC detector is placed directly below the cassette in mammography to minimize OID (in x-ray imaging, the AEC detector is most often placed above the cassette). Because radiation has to pass through the breast before reaching the detector, the primary reason for backup time and inadequate exposure is the inability of low-energy photons to penetrate the breast. *(Carlton, p. 573)*

69. **(B)** The decline in breast cancer mortality is a result of improvement in breast cancer treatment and the benefits of mammography screening. Although there is no guarantee that all patients will survive, the long-term survival rates are actually improving because cancers discovered at an earlier stage have a better prognosis, giving women a better long-term survival rate. *(ACS, p. 6)*

70. **(C)** Contaminated developer can cause wet films, an increase in the base fog, or decreased film speed. Increased contrast is likely to be caused by the developer temperature being too high, the replenishment rates being too high, or improper mixing of the developer solution. *(Andolina, pp. 96–99; Bushong, p. 322)*

71. **(B)** Spot compression increases compression to the area of suspected abnormality, allowing the tissue to spread more evenly and eliminating pseudomasses. Because of the need to reduce extraneous light (increase visualization of breast tissue), coned collimated views are no longer taken when imaging with spot compression. *(Andolina, p. 239)*

72. **(B)** The FB or caudal-cranial projection may be useful in nonconforming patients or finding lesions high on the chest wall. In performing the FB, the image receptor is above the breast and compression is applied at the inframammary fold. *(Andolina, p. 197)*

73. **(B)** If the patient stands away from the image receptor and bends forward, her chest will be brought forward and derriere back, removing the abdomen from the imaging area. If this does not achieve the desired results and the abdomen still protrudes, the mammographer cannot sacrifice posterior and lateral tissue to image the anterior breast. Two views may be required—a lateral of the anterior breast and the MLO for the posterior and upper-outer quadrant of the breast. *(Andolina, p. 251; Wentz, p. 83)*

74. **(B)** Spot compression increases compression over the area of interest, spreading out the tissue more evenly and allowing visualization of the margins or borders of lesions. Biopsy is a surgical procedure. Aspiration is generally done to check for solid versus cystic lesions, and stereotactic localization is used to localize nonpalpable lesions. Mammography is the first line of defense against breast cancer. Before further testing is undertaken, as much information on the lesion should be gathered from mammography. *(Andolina, p. 314; Wentz, p. 71)*

75. **(A)** The specimen should always be compressed and radiographed to ensure that the lesion was completely removed. If there are calcifications present, the lesion should be magnified to ensure that all the calcifications were removed. *(Andolina, p. 319; Wentz, p. 90)*

76. **(D)** Digital images will never appear too light or dark because digital imaging has the advantage of being able to manipulate the final image. In digital imaging, if a graph of the optical density (called the signal) and the relative exposure is plotted the relationship is not the H & D curve; rather, it is a straight line (Figure 6–11). The digital image therefore has a much wider latitude than conventional mammography. This ability to adjust the final image (thus reducing the need for repeats) is one of the greatest advantages of digital imaging. The problem is that, although overexposure can be corrected, the patient dose is high. The technologist encounters problems with underexposed images, however. If the digital signal is not enough to produce a "good" image, the image appears excessively noisy (appearance similar to quantum mottle). *(Andolina, pp. 444–447; Bushong, p. 317)*

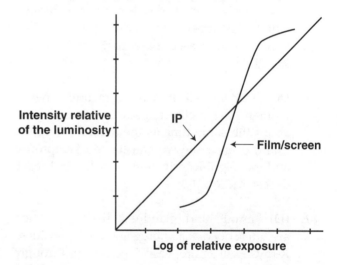

Figure 6–11. H & D curve from film-screen versus digital imaging. A graph of the optical density signal and the relative exposure for a digital imaging plate (IP) has a linear response to x-ray. This is unlike the curvilinear response of a film-screen system.

77. **(B)** Gynecomastia is a benign proliferation of tissue in the male breast. It is often seen bilaterally but can be unilateral. Gynecomastia is not associated with increased risk for breast cancer in males. *(Andolina, p. 158)*

78. **(C)** The Montgomery glands are seen as protrusions on the surface of the areola. They are

actually specialized sweat glands that usually become more prominent during pregnancy and lactation. *(Andolina, p. 140; Harris, p. 4)*

79. (A) Extended processing extends the time the film spends in the developer solution. It may also raise the temperature of the developer solution. The overall effect of extended processing is to increase the speed and contrast of some single emulsion films. The film requires less exposure; therefore, the radiation dose to the patient is lowered. *(Andolina, p. 100)*

80. (C) The humidity level in the darkroom should be between 30% and 50%. Low humidity (less than 30%) causes static and high humidity (over 50%) causes clumping of the film emulsion from water vapor clinging to the film. Dirty rollers may cause scratches on the films. Changes in developer temperature, improperly mixed developer, or contaminated developer can cause reduced film speed or increased base fog. *(Andolina, pp. 96–99)*

81. (A) Over age 40, it is recommended that a woman have a clinical breast examination at about the same time as the annual mammogram, even if the woman has no symptoms and no significantly higher risk for breast cancer. *(ACR, p. 10)*

82. (D) Fibrous and glandular tissue together are described as fibroglandular densities. X-rays will more easily penetrate through fatty tissue than through fibrous or glandular tissue. Fatty areas appear as radiolucent (black or less dense) areas on the mammogram. The fibroglandular tissue is more radiopaque than fatty tissues and results in areas of lower optical density on the mammogram (white or denser areas). *(Andolina, p. 150; Wentz, p. 12)*

83. (C) Compression decreases the thickness of the breast, bringing the breast closer to the film and increasing contrast. Resolution affects the image appearance by demonstrating fine detail of structures. Because resolution improves when the OID decreases, compres-

sion also increases spatial resolution. *(Carlton, pp. 403, 583)*

84. (D) A core biopsy removes a cylinder of tissue using a 14-gauge needle. The sample from a core biopsy is larger than that from FNA. Tissue samples from a core biopsy are assessed histologically. FNA or fine needle aspiration cytology (FNAC) is more difficult to perform. A 20- to 23-gauge needle is used to remove cellular material for cytologic analysis. Excisional biopsy is a surgical biopsy where the entire lesion as well as surrounding margins of normal-appearing tissue is removed. A wire localization is a procedure during which nonpalpable lesions or calcifications in the breast are identified by placing a thin needle into the breast. The needle is guided using mammograms or ultrasound, and a small hook wire is placed to mark the site of the lesion before surgery. *(Andolina, p. 332; Breast Cancer Resource Center: Benign Breast Conditions, p. 5)*

85. (D) The RM or RL are both useful in separating glandular structures of the breast to clear questions of superimposition. The ID projection is used in imaging augmented breast clear of the implants. The MLO is a routine projection and would not be used as an additional projection. The XCCL is best for imaging the posterolateral parts of the breast. *(Andolina, p. 269)*

86. (C) The high image receptor unnecessarily elevates the shoulder, pulling breast tissue from view but not compromising compression of the lower breast. If, however, the patient has a protruding abdomen the compression paddle will hit the abdomen, compressing the abdomen and not the lower breast. If too much shoulder muscle and axilla are allowed in the compression field, the axilla will be compressed but the thickness of the axilla will not allow for compression of the lower breast. *(Andolina, p. 198)*

87. **(C)** As a woman ages, declining hormone levels affect both the breast stroma and epithelium. The breast loses its supporting structure to fat, producing a smaller breast or a larger, more pendulous breast because of the loss of the epithelial structures and stroma. The duct system remains but the lobules shrink and collapse. This process generally begins at menopause and may continue for 3–5 years. It is referred to as *atrophy* or *involution*. Increased estrogen or hormone levels, which occur during menstruation, result in an increase in breast stroma and epithelium leading to denser breast tissue. *(Andolina, p. 153; Harris, p. 12)*

88. **(D)** The ACS suggests that breasts be examined by palpating in a circular, up-and-down, or wedge pattern, using the pads of the three middle fingers. These are the most effective means of feeling for lumps in the breast. *(Breast Cancer Resource Center: Detection and Symptoms, p. 3)*

89. **(A)** X-rays interact primarily with the entrance surface of the screen. If the screen is between the x-ray tube and the film, the excess screen blur will cause increased spatial resolution. With the film between the x-ray tube and the screen (the film is placed with the emulsion side to the screen), screen bloom is reduced and spatial resolution is improved. *(Bushong, pp. 210, 316)*

90. **(B)** Although grids increase contrast, in magnification mammography the large OID or air gap acts like a grid in reducing scatter radiation from reaching the film. Grid use in magnification would increase exposure times, increase tube loading, and thus increase motion artifact due to long exposure times. Patient radiation dose is also increased. *(ACR, p. 59; Andolina, p. 63)*

91. **(D)** The FB best visualizes the central and medial abnormalities high on the chest wall and can be done for all these reasons. The beam is directed inferiorly to superiorly. *(ACR, p. 68; Andolina, p. 194; Wentz, p. 64)*

92. **(D)** The ML provides a true representation of the breast structures in relation to the nipple, but should not be used as a routine projection because it is poor at visualizing the posterior and lateral aspects of the breast. *(Andolina, p. 219)*

93. **(D)** A request for the nipple in profile may be needed for proper measurement for needle localization or a suspected subareolar abnormality. However, putting the nipple in profile is sometimes counterproductive. Breast tissue will be lost either superiorly, inferiorly, laterally, or medially, depending on the projection and location of the nipple on the breast. Missed tissue will then lead to undetected breast cancer. If the nipple is not in profile, additional films are needed, but the original should not be discarded. *(Andolina, p. 183; Wentz, p. 79)*

94. **(B)** If the processor does not have an internal digital thermometer, any regular digital thermometer can be used. The mercury-in-glass thermometers are easily broken and will damage or contaminate the processor. Even small amounts of mercury will permanently contaminate the processor. *(Andolina, p. 112; ACR, p. 130)*

95. **(A)** Mammography units generally have two sets of focal spot sizes, one for routine imaging and the other for magnification. To maintain a sharp image during magnification, a small focal spot size is used. The small focal spot size increases resolution. Resolution is also increased by decreasing the thickness of the part under compression, thereby lessening geometric unsharpness. *(Carlton, p. 582)*

96. **(A)** The HVL of the x-ray beam is that thickness of absorbing material needed to reduce the intensity of the beam to half of its original value. Dosimeter equipment and an ionization chamber are just two of a number of methods that can be used to measure the radiation intensity for successively thicker sections of filters. The slit camera is generally the most effective measuring tool used to determine the focal spot size. The star pattern

and the pinhole camera can also be used to measure focal spot size. *(Andolina, p. 12; Bushong, p. 431)*

97. **(A)** The overall repeat rate should be approximately 2% or less, but a rate of 5% is probably adequate. If the repeat rate exceeds the acceptable level (2% or 5%) or if repeat or reject rates change from the previously measured rate by more than ±2%, the change should be investigated and corrective action taken. *(ACR, p. 207)*

98. **(C)** Oil cysts show mammographically as high-density tumors with lucent centers and eggshell-like calcifications. They usually form as a result of fat necrosis or are calcified hematomas. Fat necrosis is death of fatty tissue in the breast that can occur spontaneously, but is usually the result of a biopsy or injury. When the fat tissue dies, it changes to oil. The body then forms a capsule around the oil to protect itself. The capsule generally has a thin layer of calcifications, which give an eggshell-like appearance on the mammogram. Oil cysts are benign. Ductal papillomas are benign masses associated with the ducts and are not seen mammographically. A fibroadenoma is a benign radiolucent mass that may or may not contain calcifications. A hematoma is seen as a circular-oval lesion with mixed density. It is a benign mass associated with injury or surgery. *(Andolina, p. 158; Tabár, pp. 28, 199)*

99. **(C)** The final mammographic image should be evaluated under ideal viewing conditions. Excellent viewing conditions include low ambient room light to minimize light reflected off the surface of the film. The viewboxes should be cleaned and checked regularly because they can become dirty or the luminance of the bulbs can fade. Masking films eliminates viewbox light, which has not passed through the exposed area of the film, from reaching the eye. If the extraneous viewbox light is blocked, it is often possible to see the skin and subcutaneous tissues. *(ACR, p. 92; Wentz, p. 51)*

100. **(C)** The ID projection is a modified compression technique for imaging the augmented breast. The method displaces the implant posteriorly to exclude it from the compression area. ID projections are taken in addition to the routine projections. In general, the routine series for a patient with breast augmentation would be routine CC (both breasts), routine MLO (both breasts), CC with ID (both breasts), and MLO with ID (both breasts). *(Andolina, p. 227)*

101. **(D)** Under the final FDA regulations, all technologists satisfying the interim regulations can still perform mammograms. All new technologists performing mammograms must:

   - complete at least 40 contact hours of documented training in mammography under the supervision of a qualified instructor or, before April 28, 1999, have satisfied the requirements of the interim regulation of the FDA
   - perform a minimum of 25 examinations under direct supervision of a qualified technologist
   - have at least 8 hours of training in each mammography modality in which the techologist intends to practice (for example, digital versus conventional screen–film systems) if the technologist started working in the new modality after April 28, 1999.

   (Accreditation and Certification Overview: Technologist Training)

102. **(B)** For proper positioning of the MLO, the pectoral muscle is wide superiorly with a convex anterior border, extending to or below the posterior nipple line. Other criteria include that there is no evidence of motion and deep and superficial tissues are well separated. *(ACR, p. 42)*

103. **(A)** Ductal ectasia is a benign inflammatory condition of the ducts, which leads to nipple discharge, nipple inversion, or periareola sepsis. The condition may resemble breast carcinoma. Paget's disease of the breast is a special form of ductal carcinoma associated

with changes of the nipple. Peau d'orange is a condition where the skin of the breast becomes thickened and dimpled, resembling an orange; this may be the result of either benign or malignant conditions. Ductal papillomas are benign masses associated with the ducts and are not usually seen mammographically. *(Tabár, pp. 2, 199, 241; Thomas, p. 582)*

104. **(A)** In the immature breast the ducts and alveoli are lined by a two-layer epithelium of cells. After puberty this epithelium proliferates, forming three alveolar cell types: superficial (luminal) A cells, basal B cells (chief cells), and myoepithelial cells. Beneath the epithelium is connective tissue that helps to keep the epithelium in place. Between the epithelium and the connective tissue is a layer called the basement membrane. *(Harris, p. 10; Tortora, pp. 105, 1000)*

105. **(B)** In this form of unsharpness there is a further spread of light from the screen before it reaches the film. Unlike motion unsharpness, which covers a wider area, unsharpness due to poor screen contact is usually localized. Noisy images are mainly due to scatter or quantum mottle. When not enough photons are used to form the image, the result is a greater amount of quantum mottle. Image contrast refers to the variations of tissue density seen on the image. *(ACR, pp. 104–105)*

106. **(B)** Mammoplasty is the reshaping of the breast. The breast can be lifted to reduce a sagging breast, enlarged (augmented), or reconstructed after the removal of a tumor. Reduction mammoplasty is the term used to describe the reduction of the size of the breast by removing excess breast tissue. A breast biopsy is the removal of breast tissue for histologic testing. *(Thomas, p. 1158)*

107. **(B)** Quantum mottle is one of the principal causes of radiographic noise. Radiographic noise is the undesirable fluctuation in the density of the image due to fluctuations in the number of x-ray photons interacting with the image receptor. The quantum mottle will be higher if the x-rays are produced with few x-ray photons. Film graininess is the distribution in size and space of the silver halide grains in the emulsion, and resolution refers to the ability to visually detect separate objects distinct from each other. Motion results in blurring unsharpness of the image. *(ACR, pp. 102–105; Bushong, p. 254)*

108. **(C)** Yellow brown stains on the film are caused by thiosulfate from the fixer, left on the film because of improper washing. This generally indicates a problem with hyporetention from the fixer. The silver sulfide slowly builds up and appears as yellow in the stored radiograph. Streaks on the film can result from light leaks in the cassette; a round spot of increased density may be due to low humidity (static). Areas of reduced density could be caused by pressure on the film before exposure. *(Bushong, pp. 445–446)*

109. **(C)** In the SIO projection the beam is directed from the superolateral to the inferomedial surface of the breast; therefore, the medial breast is closest to the image recorder. *(Andolina, p. 208)*

110. **(D)** In general, male breast imaging will present the same difficulty as imaging a small, dense female breast and the breast size of males is sometimes no different than that of females. However, because of chest hair on males, the breast tends to slip from under the compression. *(Andolina, p. 253)*

111. **(D)** In the SIO the rays are directed from the lateral portion of the upper axilla to the lower medial portion of the breast, that is, superiolateral to inferomedial. The superomedial to inferolateral is the routine MLO and the inferolateral to superomedial is the LMO. The inferomedial to superolateral has no ACR label. *(Andolina, pp. 180, 208)*

112. **(B)** Under current regulations, an accreditation body can be a private, non-profit organization or state agency. Currently, the FDA-approved accreditation bodies are the ACR and the states of Arkansas, California, Iowa, and Texas. Accreditation bodies can accredit

only those facilities located within their respective states. *(Accreditation and Certification Overview)*

113. **(B)** The MLO is one of the routine imaging projections. The reverse of this is the LMO. This projection will give a mirror image of the MLO and is useful in imaging patients with pacemakers. The LMO and also the LM are good alternatives to the routine images and both can also be used for patients with infusa-port (port-a-caths inserted for long-term chemotherapy treatment), the kyphotic patient, and patients with recent open-heart surgery. The ML is not a good replacement because it is poor at imaging the posterior and lateral aspects of the breast. The XCCL only images the posterolateral breast tissue. *(Andolina, pp. 191, 217)*

114. **(D)** In breast localization the shortest skin-to-abnormality distance should always be used unless that projection will not demonstrate the abnormality. In addition to these reasons, the greater the distance the needle travels in the breast, the greater the risk of deflection. *(Andolina, p. 393)*

115. **(D)** These are MQSA requirements. The assessment of findings refers to the final result (for example, benign). Additional patient identifiers could be the patient's age, date of birth, or medical record number. *(Accreditation and Certification Overview: Record Keeping)*

CHAPTER 7

Practice Test 2
Questions

1. Radiation therapy is a treatment that utilizes

   (A) drugs to treat cancer that may have spread
   (B) high-energy radiation to destroy cancer cells
   (C) radioactive tracers to track the path of cancer to the lymph nodes
   (D) potent pain medication to treat the severe pain from cancer

2. Between ages 20 and 30 an asymptomatic woman should be having a mammogram every

   (A) year
   (B) 2 years
   (C) 3 years
   (D) none of the above

3. Medical history may include questions on contraceptive use because

   (A) synthetic hormones such as contraceptives are known to cause breast cancer
   (B) reproductive hormones are a factor in breast cancer
   (C) family history of hormone use predisposes a woman to cancer
   (D) personal history of hormone use decreases a woman's risk for breast cancer

4. X-ray photons leaving the breast enter the top of the cassette

   1. to go through the intensifying screen before reaching the film
   2. then go through the film before reaching the intensifying screen
   3. react with the single intensifying screen of the cassette

   (A) 1 and 2
   (B) 2 and 3
   (C) 1 and 3
   (D) 1, 2, and 3

5. In quality control, if your data consistently exceeds the operating level you need to

   (A) establish new operating limits
   (B) narrow the control limits
   (C) widen the control limits
   (D) repair or replace equipment

6. A control film crossover should be carried out

   (A) whenever the processing chemistry is changed
   (B) when a new box of film is opened
   (C) if a new processor is installed
   (D) if the control limits consistently exceed the normal values

7. In digital imaging a graph of the density range to the log of relative exposure (the characteristic curve or H & D curve used in conventional imaging) shows a

   (A) shallow sloping curve
   (B) steep sloping curve
   (C) linear response
   (D) curve similar to conventional imaging

8. On the ACR approved accreditation phantom the total number of fibers, speck groups, and masses is

   (A) 5 fibers, 5 speck groups, and 5 masses
   (B) 5 fibers, 6 speck groups, and 5 masses
   (C) 6 fibers, 5 speck groups, and 5 masses
   (D) 5 fibers, 5 speck groups, and 6 masses

9. The circular pigmented area around the nipple is called the

   (A) skin
   (B) areola
   (C) Montgomery gland
   (D) ampulla

10. A wart is demonstrated mammographically as a

    (A) sharply outlined multilobulated lesion
    (B) sharply outlined lesion with a halo
    (C) mixed-density circular lesion with a radiolucent center
    (D) mixed-density oval lesion

11. Figure 7–1 indicates

    (A) mammographically benign calcifications
    (B) malignant calcifications
    (C) warts
    (D) fibroadenomas

12. What immediate action reduces motion unsharpness in compression mammography?

    (A) Compression reduces breast thickness
    (B) Compression immobilizes the breast
    (C) Compression brings the image closer to the image receptor
    (D) Compression reduces scatter and improves contrast

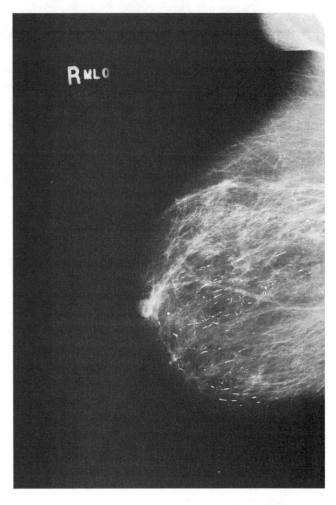

Figure 7–1.

13. In magnification, what immediate role does the large OID play in reducing scattered radiation?

    (A) Most of the scattered radiation misses the image receptor
    (B) Exposure is reduced because a grid is not needed
    (C) The compressed breast allows lower kVp values
    (D) The larger SID utilizes the inverse square law

14. Quantum mottle on the film is reduced by

    (A) high kVp
    (B) high mAs
    (C) motion
    (D) fast intensifying screens

15. What is the best placement for the needle-wire during a needle localization?

    (A) The needle-wire should be immediately below the lesion
    (B) The needle-wire should be immediately above the lesion
    (C) The needle-wire should pass through the lesion
    (D) The needle-wire should pass 1 cm above lesion

16. Although it often means losing some of the lateral breast tissue, in imaging for the CC projection, most experts advise a slight medial rotation of the patient's body to include the medial breast tissue. Why?

    (A) Medial breast is imaged best on the CC
    (B) Medial breast is imaged only on the CC
    (C) Lateral breast is distorted on the CC
    (D) The slight medial rotation enables ease in positioning

17. Which is true for all TAN positioning?

    (A) The patient is always in the CC position
    (B) The central ray is always directed vertically
    (C) The central ray is always parallel to the plane of the breast
    (D) The central ray is always perpendicular to the skin surface

18. In the RRM position, the lower section of the breast is rolled in which direction?

    (A) Laterally
    (B) Medially
    (C) Inferiorly
    (D) Superiorly

19. A radiolucent implant used in breast reconstruction is the

    (A) saline implant
    (B) TRAM flap implant
    (C) silicone liquid implant
    (D) silicone gel implant

20. In addition to the routine CC and MLO, a routine series for a postmastectomy patient would also include the

    (A) AT
    (B) ML
    (C) TAN
    (D) LMO

21. Men with a family history of breast cancer have

    (A) a greater risk for breast cancer
    (B) a minor risk for breast cancer
    (C) no significantly increased risk for breast cancer
    (D) a personal history of breast cancer

22. The CBE should be performed

    (A) at or near the time of the annual mammogram
    (B) only by the radiologist
    (C) monthly, preferable at the same time of the month
    (D) at least twice a year

23. The absorbed dose in mammography is generally _____ the entrance skin exposure (ESE).

    (A) significantly higher than
    (B) significantly lower than
    (C) about the same as
    (D) higher in a small breast than

24. The MQSA requires that the maximum compression for the initial power drive not exceed

    (A) 100 Newtons
    (B) 200 Newtons
    (C) 400 Newtons
    (D) 500 Newtons

25. Collimation should not extend beyond any edge of the image receptor by more than

    (A) 1% of the SID
    (B) 2% of the SID
    (C) 3% of the SID
    (D) 4% of the SID

26. The characteristic curve of a particular film describes the relationship between the

    (A) exposure the film receives and the density after processing
    (B) x-ray beam quality of the mammographic unit and film speed
    (C) speed of the film and the density at different exposure levels
    (D) screen-film combination as it relates to the selected mAs

27. Under which of the following circumstances is it necessary to reestablish processor QC operating levels?

    (A) A change in film volume
    (B) A change in mammographer
    (C) An unexplained upward change in the data
    (D) Using a different sensitometer

28. Given the density inside the disc = 1.23; the mid-density = 1.25; the background density = 1.68; the density adjacent to the disc = 1.66; and the highest density = 1.69, what is the density difference on the phantom image?

    (A) 0.42
    (B) 0.43
    (C) 0.44
    (D) 0.45

29. Breast tissue can extend medially to the

    (A) latissimus dorsi muscle
    (B) midsternum
    (C) retromammary space
    (D) inframammary crease

30. Which of the following hormones has the most influence on the normal physiologic changes of the breast?

    1. Prolactin
    2. Estrogen
    3. Progesterone

        (A) 1 and 2 only
        (B) 2 and 3 only
        (C) 1 and 3 only
        (D) 1, 2, and 3

31. Which of the following is (are) considered a first-degree relative?

    1. mother
    2. aunt
    3. sister

        (A) 1 only
        (B) 1 and 2 only
        (C) 2 and 3 only
        (D) 1 and 3 only

32. A woman should perform BSE monthly to

    (A) become familiar with both of her breasts
    (B) localize cancerous lumps
    (C) recognize breast dimpling
    (D) discover the best method of BSE

33. The breast of a woman under age 35 is

    (A) not related to radiation sensitivity
    (B) less sensitive to radiation
    (C) less sensitive to low-dose radiation
    (D) more sensitive to radiation

34. In the low kVp range using a molybdenum target tube, what type of photon interaction predominates?

    (A) Photoelectric interaction
    (B) Compton interactions
    (C) Bremsstrahlung interaction
    (D) Coherent interaction

35. In digital imaging a repeat analysis test is

    (A) unnecessary—digital automatically corrects exposure mistakes
    (B) necessary—digital cannot correct for overexposure
    (C) unnecessary—digital corrects unsharpness by altering the spatial display
    (D) necessary—digital cannot correct motion unsharpness

36. The same mammographer should view the phantom images because

    (A) subjective judgment about images is always difficult
    (B) it is not wise to have different individuals handling the phantom
    (C) not all mammographers know the MQSA regulations
    (D) different mammographers will calculate the optical density differently

37. The FB projection utilizes a beam directed

    (A) perpendicular to the image recorder
    (B) horizontally
    (C) tangentially
    (D) parallel to the image recorder

38. Radiation changes that the breast may exhibit include

    1. erythema
    2. edema
    3. hardening

       (A) 1 and 2
       (B) 2 and 3
       (C) 1 and 3
       (D) 1, 2, and 3

39. Magnification in mammography can be useful in all of the following EXCEPT

    (A) specimen radiographs
    (B) to define borders of masses
    (C) to assess calcification
    (D) routine screening

40. Which of the following projections could be used to replace the MLO in patients where the MLO is not possible?

    (A) ML
    (B) LM
    (C) RM
    (D) AT

41. A papilloma is a

    (A) benign lesion in the nipple
    (B) malignant lesion in the nipple
    (C) benign lesion in the ducts
    (D) malignant lesion in the ducts

42. The best time for a woman to perform a BSE is

    (A) before the start of the monthly period
    (B) just after the period starts
    (C) 7–10 days after the start of the period
    (D) anytime

43. It may be necessary to use manual technique with small breast because the

    (A) multiple detectors can be moved according to breast size
    (B) AEC detector may not cover the small breast tissue area
    (C) AEC detector cannot compensate for breast size
    (D) AEC cannot compensate for varying breast tissue types

44. If an artifact is noted on some mammographic images, which appropriate MQSA regulation will identify the dirty cassette quickly and easily?

    (A) Processor quality control test
    (B) Screen cleanliness
    (C) Visual checklist
    (D) Standardized image labeling

45. Which of the following tests are performed monthly?

    (A) Phantom images
    (B) Repeat/reject analysis
    (C) Compression check
    (D) Visual checklist

46. On a reject/repeat analysis, the rate was lower than 5% but one category of the reject/repeat analysis is significantly higher than others. What should be done?

    (A) Although the overall rate is under 5%, the one area should be targeted for improvement

    (B) If the other categories are within normal limits that area can be disregarded

    (C) Because the rate was over 2% the entire department needs to be reassessed

    (D) With a overall rate lower than 5% one high rate is statistically meaningless

47. Typically, grid ratios in mammography range from

    (A) 7:1 to 8:1
    (B) 6:1 to 8:1
    (C) 3:1 to 6:1
    (D) 3:1 to 5:1

48. Positron emission tomography (PET) imaging is useful in staging tumors because

    (A) the positron-emitting isotopes are radioactive

    (B) PET imaging can display an image of the tumor bed

    (C) the positron-emitting isotopes destroy the tumor bed

    (D) PET imaging tracks the increased blood flow from the cancerous tumor

49. Medical history is important in

    1. assessing risk factors for breast cancer
    2. preventing breast cancer
    3. evaluating treatment options

    (A) 1 and 2 only
    (B) 2 and 3 only
    (C) 1 and 3 only
    (D) 1, 2, and 3

50. Unlike conventional tubes, some mammography tubes are tilted 7.5–12° from the horizontal. The effect of this is to

    1. allow the use of smaller focal spot size
    2. minimize the heel effect
    3. increase resolution

    (A) 1 and 2 only
    (B) 2 and 3 only
    (C) 1 and 3 only
    (D) 1, 2, and 3

51. The retromammary space describes the area

    (A) between the breast and pectoral muscle

    (B) separating the skin of the breast from the deep fascia

    (C) separating the skin from the superficial fascia

    (D) between the glandular tissue and the inframammary fold

52. In which of the following are breast cysts more common?

    1. Young women in their early 20s
    2. Premenopausal woman
    3. Postmenopausal woman on estrogen therapy

    (A) 1 and 2 only
    (B) 2 and 3 only
    (C) 1 and 3 only
    (D) 1, 2, and 3

53. The CC shows a circumscribed oval radiolucent lesion. There was a definite halo surrounding the lesion. It is most likely to be a

    (A) fibroadenoma
    (B) lymph nodes
    (C) cyst
    (D) hematoma

54. What effect does compression have on Compton interactions?

    (A) The absolute number of Compton interactions increases
    (B) The absolute number of Compton interactions decreases
    (C) Compression has no affect on Compton interactions
    (D) Compression affects Compton interaction only above 70 kVp

55. Visual inspection done during CBE involves

    (A) feeling for changes in the breast
    (B) looking for changes in the breast
    (C) palpating the breast
    (D) examining areas under the armpit

56. If the residual hypo in the mammography film exceeds $0.05 \, \text{g/m}^2$ or $5 \, \mu\text{g/cm}^2$ this indicates

    1. improper washing of the film
    2. improper fixer replenishment
    3. the film will have poor archival quality

    (A) 1 and 2 only
    (B) 2 and 3 only
    (C) 1 and 3 only
    (D) 1, 2, and 3

57. Fatty tissue is generally radiolucent and will show on the mammogram as

    (A) glandular areas
    (B) high-density areas
    (C) low-density areas
    (D) medium-density areas

58. The mammogram of a woman age 50 who has recently started estrogen replacement therapy is likely to be

    (A) more fibroglandular than her past mammographic study
    (B) more fatty that her previous mammogram
    (C) less fibrous and less glandular than her previous studies
    (D) unchanged from her previous mammograms

59. The mammogram shows an oval-shaped lesion with mixed density. The lesion has a central radiolucent area and is freely movable. This lesion is most likely to be a

    (A) fibroadenoma
    (B) hematoma
    (C) lymph node
    (D) galactocele

60. If a cyst moves down on the ML from its position on the MLO, the cyst is located

    (A) centrally
    (B) medially
    (C) laterally
    (D) at the areola

61. Increased OID causes loss of image detail in magnification mammography. What factors help to compensate for this loss of image detail?

    1. Compression of the part
    2. Decreased focal spot size
    3. Increased OID

    (A) 1 and 2 only
    (B) 2 and 3 only
    (C) 1 and 3 only
    (D) 1, 2, and 3

62. What does the actual focal spot size measure?

    (A) The area on the anode exposed to electrons
    (B) The area projected on the patient
    (C) The area projected on the image recorder
    (D) The nominal focal spot size

63. Men have a much lower risk of developing breast cancer and account for about _____ of breast cancer incidence and mortality in America.

    (A) 1%
    (B) 2%
    (C) 3%
    (D) 4%

64. The density difference on the sensitometric strip is the difference between

    (A) the average density closest to 2.20 and the mid-density
    (B) the mid-density and the base plus fog
    (C) the average density closest to 0.45 and the mid-density
    (D) the high and low average densities

65. What is epithelial hyperplasia?

    (A) A calcified hematoma resulting from trauma
    (B) An oil cyst within the breast
    (C) An overgrowth of cells in the ducts or lobules
    (D) A sebaceous cyst in the oil glands of the skin

66. Figure 7–2 shows a (an)

    (A) ruptured implant
    (B) encapsulated implant
    (C) herniated implant
    (D) implant removal

Figure 7–2.

67. After a four-view mammogram, calcifications are visualized superior to the nipple but only on the MLO projection. What additional projection would BEST be used to locate the position of the lesion?

    (A) XCCL
    (B) CV
    (C) ML
    (D) AX

68. Approximately how much contrast is injected into the breast during ductography?

    (A) 1–5 cc
    (B) 15–25 cc
    (C) 30–40 cc
    (D) 50–100 cc

69. What does the glandular dose measure?

    (A) The average dose to the patient's skin
    (B) The absorbed dose to the skin
    (C) The absorbed dose to the tissue
    (D) The same as the entrance skin dose

70. Which of the following relationships does NOT change when moving from routine to magnification mammography?

    (A) OID
    (B) Focal spot size
    (C) SID
    (D) SOD

71. Who performs the compression device check for mammography QC?

    (A) Physicist
    (B) Staff technologist
    (C) Radiologist
    (D) Mammographer

72. A galactocele is

    (A) a lesion associated with trauma to the breast
    (B) a benign milk-filled cyst
    (C) associated with shell-like calcification
    (D) associated with a central radiolucent hilus

73. During pregnancy and lactation the breast

    (A) shows increased density
    (B) increases in fatty content
    (C) atrophies
    (D) shows decreased density

74. Most of the glandular tissue is arranged in the breast around the

    (A) medial and upper-inner quadrants
    (B) lateral and lower-inner quadrants
    (C) central and upper-outer quadrants
    (D) medial and upper-outer quadrants

75. A beryllium (Be) window enhances contrast by

    (A) increasing the output of the x-ray tube
    (B) reducing production of scattered radiation
    (C) transmitting more low-energy photons
    (D) transmitting more high-energy photons

76. Proper compression of the breast is indicated when the

    (A) patient is in pain
    (B) compression paddle stops
    (C) breast is taut
    (D) breast feels soft

77. Which factors cause increased skin dose in magnification?

    1. Larger OID
    2. Smaller focal spot size
    3. Increased mAs

    (A) 1 and 2 only
    (B) 2 and 3 only
    (C) 1 and 3 only
    (D) 1, 2, and 3

78. In radiology, according to the line focus principle, the effective focal spot is

    (A) larger than the actual focal spot
    (B) smaller than the actual focal spot
    (C) the same as the actual focal spot
    (D) decreased as the target angle increases

79. A palpable lesion, highly suspicious for malignancy, is seen in the CC and MLO of the left breast during routine mammography. The borders are highly irregular. The next test could be

    (A) stereostatic localization
    (B) needle localization
    (C) ductography
    (D) core biopsy

80. In the optimum position of the patient for the CC projection, the patient's head is turned

    (A) toward the side under examination
    (B) away from the side under examination
    (C) depending on the preference of the technologist
    (D) to the patient's right

81. Which of the following projections would best separate superimposed 12 o'clock and 6 o'clock masses?

    (A) MLO
    (B) XCCL
    (C) CC
    (D) AT

82. The positioning terminology CV means

    (A) compressed view
    (B) Cleopatra view
    (C) cleavage view
    (D) compression view

83. Malignant casting-type calcifications appear on the mammogram as

    (A) granulated sugar or crushed stone calcifications
    (B) eggshell-like calcifications
    (C) elongated, branching, and needle-like calcifications
    (D) fragmented, linear branching calcifications

84. The functional milk-producing units of the breast are contained within the

(A) lactiferous sinuses

(B) lobules

(C) ampulla

(D) areola

85. If the nipple is not imaged in profile on the four-view series, indications to take additional views with the nipple in profile include

1. the nipple cannot be differentiated from a mass

2. the patient has a possible retroareolar mass

3. the patient is male

   (A) 1 and 2 only

   (B) 1 and 3 only

   (C) 2 and 3 only

   (D) 1, 2, and 3

86. The AT projection best demonstrates the

(A) subareolar area

(B) medial aspect of the breast

(C) axillary aspect of the breast

(D) lower inner quadrant of the breast

87. The area of minus-density in the upper part of Figure 7–3 best represents

(A) the patient's shoulder

(B) a pressure artifact occurring after the exposure

(C) the patient's chin

(D) malposition of the mirror supplying illumination

88. The patient had trauma to the breast 5 days ago and has developed a lump. Such an injury may show mammographically as a

(A) galactocele

(B) hematoma

(C) lymph node

(D) fibroadenoma

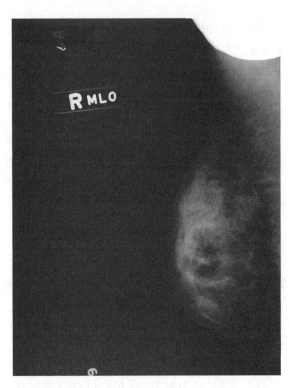

Figure 7–3.

89. Exposure factors are determined by all of the following EXCEPT

(A) the patient

(B) target material

(C) screen/film combination

(D) viewing conditions

90. If too much upper axilla and shoulder are under the compression paddle when imaging for the MLO, the effect is to

(A) inhibit proper compression of the upper breast

(B) inhibit proper compression of the lower breast

(C) ensure equal compression of the upper and lower breast

(D) ensure proper compression of the lower breast

91. Of these four, which would best demonstrate microcalcifications?

 (A) Ultrasound
 (B) Spot compression
 (C) Spot magnification
 (D) TAN projection

92. What part of the breast exhibits Paget's disease?

 (A) Nipple
 (B) Skin
 (C) Areola
 (D) Tail of Spence

93. A rolled projection can be performed to

 1. remove superimposed tissues
 2. separate superimposed breast tissue
 3. determine the location of a finding seen only on one of the standard views

 (A) 1 and 2 only
 (B) 1 and 3 only
 (C) 2 and 3 only
 (D) 1, 2, and 3

94. Ideally, when should a breast tissue specimen be imaged?

 (A) Immediately after surgery
 (B) Within 24 hours of the surgery
 (C) While the patient is still in the recovery room
 (D) Before the surgery is terminated

95. Which projection gives a mirror image of the MLO?

 (A) ML
 (B) LM
 (C) LMO
 (D) AT

96. The nominal focal spot size of the mammography unit is 0.3. This means that the

 (A) actual focal spot size is 0.3
 (B) effective focal spot size is 0.3
 (C) effective and actual focal spot size are both 0.3
 (D) actual focal spot is smaller than 0.3

97. Women with lumpectomy should have magnified views taken of the tumor bed to

 1. confirm the removal of the cancer
 2. check calcium that may result from radiation and surgical changes
 3. check for recurrence of the cancer

 (A) 1 and 2
 (B) 2 and 3
 (C) 1 and 3
 (D) 1, 2, and 3

98. A lesion is present on the MLO but is not seen on the CC projection. What projection could best be used to determine whether the lesion is laterally or medially located?

 (A) XCCL
 (B) CV
 (C) ML
 (D) AX

99. Delaying the processing of films will affect the

 1. speed of the film
 2. film contrast
 3. density of the film

 (A) 1 and 2 only
 (B) 2 and 3 only
 (C) 1 and 3 only
 (D) 1, 2, and 3

100. When imaging a small breast, scattered radiation can be minimized by

    1. increasing compression
    2. reducing kVp
    3. reducing field size

        (A) 1 and 2 only
        (B) 2 and 3 only
        (C) 1 and 3 only
        (D) 1, 2, and 3

101. The purpose of the certification and accreditation process is to

    (A) provide legal mammography services
    (B) establish minimum national quality standards for mammography
    (C) ensure that all women have access to a certified mammography facility
    (D) authorize certain states to certify mammography facilities and conduct inspections

102. A facility has a sign posted advising patients to contact a designated person within the organization with comments. This facility is meeting the FDA's

    (A) medical outcome audit program
    (B) record keeping program
    (C) patient communication of results program
    (D) customer complaint program

103. A hamartoma is

    (A) a malignant tumor of the breast
    (B) a benign tumor of the breast
    (C) associated with trauma of the breast
    (D) associated with nursing

104. After parturition, contraction of which cells help to eject milk from the alveoli?

    (A) Epithelial cells
    (B) Myoepithelial cells
    (C) Basement cells
    (D) Superficial cells

105. A finding of incomplete on the mammogram means that the mammogram

    (A) cannot accurately evaluate the breast
    (B) showed benign findings
    (C) showed suspicious findings
    (D) is suggestive for malignancy

106. Erythema of the breast generally indicates

    (A) inflammatory breast cancer
    (B) breast abscess
    (C) breast infections
    (D) further testing of the breast is necessary

107. Which of the following is used as a treatment for estrogen-dependent tumors in post- and premenopausal women?

    (A) Radiation therapy
    (B) Chemotherapy
    (C) Tamoxifen
    (D) Antibody therapy

108. Causes of radiographic noise include

    1. quantum mottle on the film
    2. scattered radiation
    3. film graininess

        (A) 1 and 2 only
        (B) 2 and 3 only
        (C) 1 and 3 only
        (D) 1, 2, and 3

109. A thin supportive layer located between the basal surface of the epithelium and the connective tissue layer of the lobule is called

    (A) chief cells
    (B) myoepithelial
    (C) basement membrane
    (D) superficial A cells

110. A "camel's nose" breast contour can be prevented in the MLO projection by

    (A) including all of the breast under the compression paddle
    (B) angling the image receptor parallel to the pectoralis muscle
    (C) properly supporting the breast during compression
    (D) ensuring that the nipple remains in profile during compression

111. The SIO will best demonstrate the

    (A) OUQ and the LOQ of the breast
    (B) LIQ and the UIQ of the breast
    (C) UIQ and LOQ of the breast
    (D) LIQ and the OUQ

112. The basic premise of a medical audit is that

    1. all positive mammograms should be followed
    2. the pathology results of all biopsies performed should be collected
    3. all pathology results should be correlated with the radiologist's findings

    (A) 1 and 2 only
    (B) 2 and 3 only
    (C) 1 and 3 only
    (D) 1, 2, and 3

113. Under the MQSA, how long are facilities required to maintain the records of a patient who died shortly after her first mammogram?

    (A) 5 years
    (B) 10 years
    (C) 20 years
    (D) Permanently

114. Under what circumstances are triangulation techniques necessary?

    1. To locate an abnormality visualized on one projection only
    2. During sterostatic breast biopsy
    3. To perform spot magnification

    (A) 1 and 2 only
    (B) 2 and 3 only
    (C) 1 and 3 only
    (D) 1, 2, and 3

115. A dimpled skin condition seen in cases of lymphatic edema of the breast is called

    (A) inflammatory carcinoma
    (B) ductal ectasia
    (C) plasma cell mastitis
    (D) peau d'orange

Answers and Explanations

1. **(B)** Many women are choosing conservation therapy that removes the tumor with wide margins (lumpectomy, quadrectomy, or segmental mastectomy) and includes radiation therapy (irradiation with high-energy beams). Treatment starts 3–8 weeks after surgery and includes about 5–6 weeks of daily treatments. *(Andolina, p. 309)*

2. **(D)** An annual mammogram is generally recommended for asymptomatic women over age 40 who have not been identified as having significantly higher risk. *(ACS, p. 11)*

3. **(B)** Studies have suggested that reproductive hormones influence breast cancer risk as well as promote cancer growth. Early menarche (less than 12 years), late menopause (equal to or more than 55 years), oral contraceptive use, and fewer pregnancies will all increase a woman's risk by affecting reproductive hormones. *(ACS, p. 9)*

4. **(B)** The intensifying screen is placed behind the film in mammography cassettes to reduce screen blur. There is high x-ray absorption by the screen phosphors closest to the film emulsion reducing the diffusion of light emitted from the screen. The result is less noise and greater spatial resolution. *(Bushong, p. 316)*

5. **(D)** If data seldom exceed the operating limits by ±0.1%, the medical physicist or radiologist may wish to narrow the control limits. If the limits are consistently exceeded, it is necessary to improve the QC procedures or repair or replace the appropriate equipment. Establishing new limits is allowed only under specific circumstances, such as if the film is changed or there are changes in processing method (equipment or solutions, for example). Widening the control limits is never allowed. *(ACR, pp. 134–135)*

6. **(B)** Whenever a new box of film is opened for QC, a crossover must be carried out. Radiographic films are produced in batches, which will have slight variations in characteristics of the film emulsion. This will affect the sensitometric characteristics of the film. The crossover is carried out only with seasoned processor chemistry that is operating within plus or minus 0.10 of the control limits. The crossover is used to compare the average density steps MD, DD, and base-plus-fog of five films from the old box with five films from the new box. The new operating level is established by adding the difference (new minus old operating values) to the old operating level. If the difference is positive, the new operating level is increased. If the difference is negative, the new operating level is decreased (Figure 7–4). If control limits consistently exceed the normal values, the equipment needs to be repaired or replaced. Whenever new equipment is installed (processor, sensitometer, or densitometer), the processor QC operating levels must be reestablished. *(ACR, p. 161)*

7. **(C)** Digital detectors have image characteristic similar to the response of screen-film except that the response in digital is linear (Figure 7–5). This means that regardless of the intensity of the x-ray beam, a small change in the intensity is recorded as the same change

New Emulsion #				24578	Old Emulsion #				23456
Film #	Low Density (LD) Step # 10	Mid Density (MD) Step # 11	High Density (HD) Step # 13	B+F	Film #	Low Density (LD) Step # 10	Mid Density (MD) Step # 11	High Density (HD) Step # 13	B+F
1	0.49	1.25	2.39	0.18	1	0.46	1.27	2.33	0.17
2	0.50	1.23	2.43	0.18	2	0.48	1.30	2.30	0.17
3	0.49	1.26	2.40	0.17	3	0.46	1.27	2.28	0.18
4	0.53	1.28	2.41	0.18	4	0.48	1.28	2.32	0.17
5	0.49	1.28	2.43	0.18	5	0.47	1.31	2.35	0.18
Average	0.50	1.26	2.41	0.18	Average	0.47	1.29	2.31	0.17
Average Density Difference: DD = HD – LD = 1.91					Average Density Difference: DD = HD – LD = 1.84				

MD difference between new and old film (New MD – Old MD)	-0.03
DD difference between new and old film (New DD – Old DD)	+0.07
B+F difference between new and old film (New – Old)	+0.01

	MD	DD	B+F
Old Operating Levels	1.34	1.9	0.17
Difference between new and old film	-0.03	+0.07	+0.01
New operating levels	1.31	1.97	0.18

Figure 7–4. The Control Film Crossover Worksheet is used to calculate the difference in the average values between the new and old boxes of film and thus determine new operating levels. If the new densities are so different from the old that the new steps will not be the best choice, then new operating levels must be reestablished using the original method of establishing processor QC operating levels. (© 1999 by the American College of Radiology in *Mammography Quality Control Manual*.)

in the electronic image. In digital imaging, this is possible because there are different devices for acquisition and display, and each can be separately optimized. Digital imaging therefore has a much wider latitude than conventional imaging. Digital imaging can enhance the contrast resolution of the final image. *(Andolina, p. 441; Carlton, p. 643)*

8. **(C)** This is the total number in each group, but the criteria for the number of objects to pass the ACR are a minimum number of 4 fibers, 3 speck groups, and 3 masses (Figure

7–6). When scoring, each fiber, speck group, or mass is counted as 1 point. Partial fibers, speck groups, or masses are counted as 0.5 point or not at all. *(ACR, p. 268)*

9. **(B)** The areola is the smooth, darkened area that surrounds the nipple. Skin covers the entire breast, and the Montgomery glands are specialized sweat glands on the areola. The ampulla is another name for the lactiferous sinus, a part of the ductal system in the internal breast anatomy. *(Andolina, p. 140; Tortora, p. 946)*

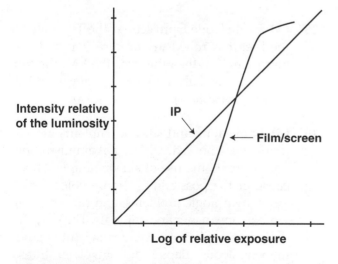

Figure 7–5. H & D curve for digital imaging. A graph of the optical density signal and the relative exposure for a digital imaging plate (IP) will have a linear response to x-ray. This is unlike the curvilinear response of a film-screen system.

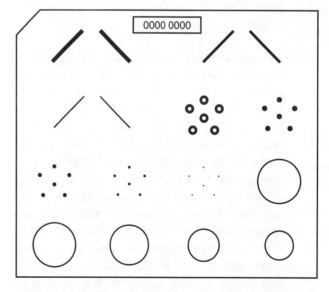

Figure 7–6. Schematic diagram of the phantom showing the relative position of the different objects embedded within the phantom.

10. **(A)** A wart forms on the skin surface of the breast and gives a typical mammographic appearance. They are multilobulated, with sharply outlined borders. An example of a mixed-density lesion with a radiolucent center is a lymph node. Other mixed-density circular or oval lesions are hematomas, galactoceles, or fibroadenolipomas. Halos are narrow radiolucent rings or ring segments around the periphery of a lesion. A halo is characteristic of benign lesions within the breast. *(Tabár, pp. 18, 48)*

11. **(A)** Plasma cell mastitis, periductal mastitis, or ductal ectasia is an inflammatory reaction characterized by the presence of plasma cells surrounding a dilated duct. It is a benign condition. Intra- and/or periductal calcifications are the final result of this condition. The calcification can be located around or inside the dilated ducts. Most are elongated and sharply outlined with smooth borders; some are needle-like with high density or may have a lucent central area. The fibroadenoma is an oval lesion that may contain calcifications. Warts rarely calcify and mammographically appear as lobulated lesions. *(Tabár, pp. 199, 209)*

12. **(B)** There are numerous advantages of compression, but the immediate action of compression in reducing motion unsharpness is immobilization. With the breast held still, the possibility of motion blur is minimized. *(Bushong, p. 314)*

13. **(A)** The large air gap acts like a grid and reduces scattered radiation, thus improving contrast. Positioning the breast away from the film takes advantage of the inverse square law: the intensity of the scattered radiation is reduced because the distance between the film and the object is increased. The SID does not change in magnification and, although a grid is not used, there is no significant reduction in exposure because of reciprocity law failure. Grid use in magnification increases exposure times, increasing tube loading, thus increasing motion artifact due to long exposure times. Patient radiation dose is also increased. *(ACR, pp. 59–60; Andolina, p. 63)*

14. **(B)** Quantum mottle refers to the mottled, grainy appearance of a radiograph. It occurs when insufficient x-rays interact with the intensifying screen to form the image. The use of high mAs, low kVp, and slower film/screen combinations reduce quantum mottle. Motion does not affect quantum mottle. *(Bushong, p. 254)*

15. **(C)** The localization needle-wire should be positioned to pass just through the lesion. Most surgeons feel for the tip of the wire before making an incision in the patient's breast. Because the tip is being used as a locator, it should be at the site of the lesion, not above or below it. *(Andolina, p. 315)*

16. **(A)** The medial breast is the most important aspect of the CC projection. The other routine projection, the MLO, often does not image medial breast clearly because of distance from the image recorder and superimposition of glandular structures. Eliminating the medial breast on the CC would therefore eliminate it from the study. *(Andolina, p. 188)*

17. **(D)** In the TAN projection, the x-ray beam just skims the area of interest. The beam is always tangential or perpendicular to the skin surface. This projection demonstrates the area of interest free of superimposition. The TAN is possible in any direction or projection. *(ACR, p. 65; Wentz, p. 70)*

18. **(A)** In the rolled projection, the top half of the breast is rolled in one direction and the bottom half in the other. For the RM, the top is rolled medially and the bottom is rolled laterally. *(Andolina, p. 239; Wentz, p. 68)*

19. **(B)** Both saline and silicone implants are radiopaque. The Federal Drug Administration now restricts the use of silicone implants because of the possibility of immunologic diseases, neurologic problems, and cancer. Most women now use saline implants. The only radiolucent implant available is the autologous myocutaneous flaps. This involves transplanting tissue from another area of the body to the breast. The most popular is the transverse rectus abdominis myocutaneous or

TRAM flap, using the rectus abdominis muscle, but the procedure can also be done using the latissimus dorsi or the gluteus maximus. Mammographically, the breast has a fatty or muscular appearance. *(Andolina, p. 306)*

20. **(B)** After mastectomy, a three-view series of CC, MLO, and ML is generally recommended. Without the other breast for comparison this three-view series gives the radiologist a better opportunity to diagnose any new malignancy. *(Andolina, p. 260)*

21. **(A)** Even though men generally have a low risk of developing breast cancer, they should be aware of the risk factors, especially family history. About 1% of males in the United States develop breast cancer each year. *(ACR, p. 8; ACS, p. 2)*

22. **(A)** The CBE is a clinical examination by a trained health care professional and should be performed every 3 years for women under 40 and every year for women over 40. To be effective the CBE should be performed in combination with a mammogram. *(ACS, p. 11)*

23. **(B)** Because of the low x-ray energies used in mammography, the dose to the skin may be high, but dose falls off rapidly as the beam penetrates the breast. The dose to the skin may be as high as 800–1000 mR/view (8–10 mGy/view); the dose to the midline of the breast (the average radiation dose to the glandular tissue or glandular dose) will be only 100 mrad (1.0 mGy). The final rules of mammography dictated by the MQSA state that a single view screen-film mammogram should not give more than 300 mrad/view average glandular dose when a grid is used and should not exceed 100 mrad/view without a grid. In diagnostic imaging, 1 R = 1 rad = 1 rem. The unit applied will depend on the specific use. *(Andolina, p. 34; Bushong, pp. 23, 553)*

24. **(B)** A compression force of a least 111 Newtons (25 lb) and a max of 200 Newtons (20 decanewtons or 45 lb) is required for the initial power drive. This is an MQSA requirement, necessary to avoid injury to patients. *(ACR, p. 201)*

25. **(B)** This is an MQSA requirement to avoid excess radiation dose to the patient. All units should have a beam-limiting device that allows the entire chest wall edge of the x-ray field to extend to the chest wall edge of the image receptor and should not extend beyond any of the edges on the image receptor by more than 2%. *(ACR, p. 109)*

26. **(A)** The characteristic curve measures the optical density or degree of blackness of the film to the log of the relative radiation exposure. A single characteristic curve can be analyzed to determine the contrast (slope of the straight-line portion of the curve) and the film latitude (the range of exposures over which the film responds with optical densities in the diagnostically useful range). Two characteristic curves of different films are needed to compare film speeds. *(Bushong, pp. 258–260)*

27. **(D)** Establishing new limits is allowed only under specific circumstances, such as if the film emulsion changes or there are changes in processing or assessment methods (new equipment or new solutions, new densitometer or sensitometer, for example). If the limits unexpectedly changed (up or down) it is necessary to improve the QC procedures or repair or replace the appropriate equipment. Widening the control limits is never allowed. *(ACR, pp. 134–135)*

28. **(B)** To determine the density difference (DD) the optical density inside the disc and density directly adjacent to the disc (to the left or right perpendicular to the anode-cathode axis) is recorded. The DD is the difference between these densities. The background density is the density measured at the center of the phantom image. The mid density and highest density are both obtained from the sensitometric strip. *(ACR, p. 167)*

29. **(B)** The breast can reach superiorly to the clavicle (level of the 2nd or 3rd rib), inferiorly to meet the abdominal wall at the level of the 6th or 7th rib (at the inframammary fold), laterally to the edge of the latissimus dorsi muscle and medially to the midsternum. *(Andolina, p. 141)*

30. **(B)** The most prominent hormones active in the breast are estrogen and progesterone. Estrogen is mostly responsible for ductal proliferation and progesterone is responsible for lobular proliferation and growth. Studies have shown the two actually work together to produce full ductal–lobular–alveolar (terminal ductules) development. Prolactin is present in the breast during initial breast growth, pregnancy, and lactation. *(Andolina, p. 146; Harris, p. 3)*

31. **(D)** First-degree relatives are immediate relatives such as mother, sister, or daughter. *(ACR, p. 8)*

32. **(A)** A woman should become familiar with both the appearance and feel of her breasts so that even small changes are noticeable. For this reason BSE should be performed regularly at the same time every month (about 1 week after a woman's period, when the breasts are least tender). *(ACS, p. 11; Breast Cancer Resource Center: Detection and Symptoms, p. 3)*

33. **(D)** Unnecessary exposure should be avoided with any radiographic examination. Some studies have shown that the dense cellular breast structure of women younger than 35 is more susceptible to radiation. *(Andolina, p. 35)*

34. **(A)** For mammography tubes made with molybdenum the most prominent x-rays are characteristic. Characteristic x-rays are produced after a photoelectric interaction. If the target is filtered with molybdenum the characteristic energy of 19 keV from the K-shell interaction will be prominent. This is within the range of energies that are most effective for mammographic imaging. Characteristic radiation is produced when an outer shell electron fills an inner shell void. If the outer shell electron fills the void in the K-shell, the x-ray emissions are termed K-characteristic x-rays. Bremsstrahlung x-rays are produced when an outer projectile electron is slowed by the electric field of the target atom nucleus. This interaction is common in tungsten targets. Coherent or classical scattering de-

scribes the interaction between low-energy electrons and atoms. The x-ray loses no energy but changes direction slightly. In Compton scattering, moderate-energy x-rays interact with an outer-shell electron and eject the electron from the atom. The ejected electron is the Compton electron. *(Bushong, pp. 165–166, 310)*

35. **(D)** Although the final testing sequence for digital has not been finalized by the MQSA, the QA testing for digital imaging will eventually have most if not all of the components of conventional imaging plus additional tests on the display and imaging system. Repeat analysis will still be needed for repeats due to positioning, patient motion, noisy images (underexposure), and equipment failure to name just a few. Digital imaging can correct for overexposure, although excessive overexposure increases the patient dose. Digital imaging has a harder time correcting for extreme underexposure, and creates a noisy image (similar to quantum mottle). Digital imaging can enhance the spatial display by enhancing the edges of spiculation or calcifications, making them more visible. Digital imaging cannot correct unsharp images, especially unsharpness due to motion. *(Andolina, pp. 248–249)*

36. **(A)** Different individuals perceive different numbers of test objects images or may count a different number of objects in the same image. For consistency, the same individual should view the images each time using the same criteria (same time of day, same viewbox, same magnifier, and same viewing conditions). The optical density calculation is a mathematical formula that does not change. *(ACR, p. 184)*

37. **(A)** The FB (from below) is the reverse craniocaudal (CC) projection. The beam is directed caudocranially to form an angle of 90° with the image recorder. *(Andolina, p. 198; Wentz, p. 64)*

38. **(D)** After radiation therapy the breast may appear red and swollen and may gradually get tighter or harden. The breast may also get smaller and be distorted from the surgical

technique. These changes are a result of the radiation and although newer radiation treatment has less effect on the breast the technologist should still handle these patients with care because the skin may be delicate and the patient may have many tender or painful areas. *(Andolina, p. 309)*

39. **(D)** Magnification is ideal for imaging small areas such as the surgical site of a patient with lumpectomy, specimen radiograph, or microcalcifications and masses. Magnification, however, should not be used for routine imaging because the entire breast may not be imaged completely and the patient dose is increased. *(Bushong, p. 316; Wentz, p. 23)*

40. **(B)** The LMO provides a mirror image of the MLO. The next best position is the LM projection, which is useful in imaging medially located lesions that are high on the chest wall or extremely posterior in the inferior half of the breast. The image on the LM is very similar to the MLO, the difference being that the MLO images the lateral portion of the breast closer to the image recorder. *(Andolina, p. 225)*

41. **(C)** Papilloma is a benign epithelial growth occurring in the larger ducts near the nipple. Generally, it produces nipple discharge. A papilloma shows only on ductography. *(Andolina, p. 158)*

42. **(C)** The best time to do the BSE is 1 week after the start of the period when the breast is least tender or swollen. If a patient is not having regular periods, the BSE should be done on the same day every month. *(Breast Cancer Resource Center: Detection and Symptoms, p. 3)*

43. **(B)** For the AEC to be effective, the thickest portion of the compressed breast, regardless of its size or tissue density, must be directly over the AEC detector. If the AEC detector does not cover the small breast tissue area the correct optical density will not record, resulting in an underpenetrated final image. *(Wentz, p. 21)*

44. **(D)** Processing control makes sure the processor is working at optimal levels. The

visual checklist verifies that the room equipment, including the mammography unit, has all the necessary accessories available and is safe for patient and technologist. Screen cleanliness ensures clean screens, but to determine which screen has the artifact all the screens would have to be opened and cleaned. Standardized image labeling identifies the mammographic unit (if there is more than one), the cassette by number, the technologist performing the examination, the patient, the facility name, and the projection. It is important to be able to identify each cassette. Dirty cassettes are thus easily identified and cleaned. *(ACR, p. 127)*

45. **(D)** Phantom images are done weekly. The repeat/reject analysis is made quarterly. Compression check is tested semiannually, and visual checks are done monthly. *(ACR, p. 119)*

46. **(A)** Ideally the rate should not exceed 2% but a rate of 5% is acceptable once a QA program has been established. An analysis of the number of repeated mammograms and rejected films identifies ways to improve efficiency and reduce cost and patient exposure. Because the main purpose of the reject/repeat analysis is to determine problem areas within the department, the one high-rate area should be targeted for improvement. *(ACR, p. 202)*

47. **(D)** The linear-type grids used in mammography typically have a very low ratio because even with a grid ratio of 4:1, patient exposure doubles (grid ratio = the height of the lead strips/the distance between the strips; ratio = h/d). Most grids are focused to the SID to increase contrast. Grids in mammography typically have a frequency of 30–50 lines per centimeter. There is a new high-transmission cellular (HTC) grid with the characteristics of a crossed grid. It can reduce scattered radiation in two directions rather than the one direction of the linear or focused grid. These grids use copper rather than lead as the grid strip, and air rather than wood or aluminum as the interspace material. When compared to a similar ratio linear grid, the HTC grids

result in equal or less radiation dose to the patient. *(Bushong, p. 315)*

48. **(B)** The staging of breast cancer is useful to determine the extent of the spread of the cancer. In general, the higher the stage of the cancer the poorer the prognosis. PET technique searches for sugar molecules that have been made radioactive and then injected into the patient. Because cancer cells grow faster than normal cells, they utilize more sugar and will accumulate the radioactive sugar particles, making the cancer's location visible with PET. The extent of the cancer is then known, which aids the oncologist in determining treatment and monitoring therapy. Currently, PET imaging is also used to differentiate recurrent cancer from treatment effects. *(Andolina, p. 414)*

49. **(C)** During the medical history, the physician collects information on the patient's risk factors for benign or malignant breast conditions and any other health problems. During the medical history session, information on past mammograms is also collected because of the importance of comparison. Although the medical history does not prevent breast cancer, it is the first step in evaluating both symptomatic and asymptomatic women and an important step in evaluating treatment options. *(ACS, pp. 8, 13; Breast Cancer Resource Center: Detection and Symptoms, p. 4)*

50. **(D)** The smaller the focal spot size, the greater the resolution; but to achieve a good resolution a small focal spot size is necessary. General radiography uses target angles of 5–15° but in mammography units the target is angled about 23° (line-focus principle). The large target angle would force the use of larger focal spot sizes and result in the heel effect (Figure 7–7). As a result of the heel effect, some of the useful beam must travel through the target material. This reduces the intensity of the useful beam at the anode end of the tube; however, with the cathode positioned to the chest wall and with the tube tilted about 6°, the central rays parallels the chest wall so no tissue is missed, the heel effect is minimized, and small focal spots are possible, resulting in increased

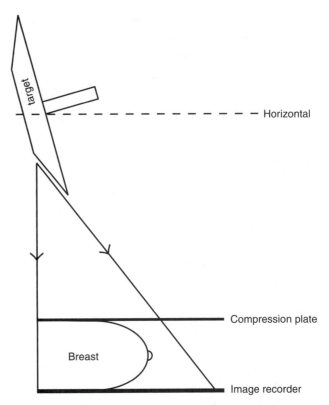

Figure 7–7. Mammography tube tilt. With the x-ray tube tilted about 6° off the horizontal the central rays run parallel to the chest wall so no breast tissue is missed. Tilting the tube allows a smaller target angle and therefore a smaller effective focal spot size while minimizing the heel effect. Tilting also allows greater anode heat capacity because the actual focal spot size is not further reduced.

resolution. The small focal spot sizes used in mammography are therefore achieved using a combination of 23° target angle and 6° tube tilt. *(Carlton, p. 570; Bushong, p. 310)*

51. **(A)** The retromammary space separates the breast from the pectoral muscle. This space is filled with a layer of adipose or fatty tissue as opposed to the supporting and connective tissue (stroma), blood vessels, and various ductal structures that make up the glandular and fibrous tissues of the breast. *(Andolina, pp. 141, 150)*

52. **(D)** Cysts occur in the terminal ductal lobular units when the extralobular terminal duct becomes blocked. Fluid accumulates faster than it can be resorbed. Cysts vary in size and respond to hormonal fluctuations, but the development of a cyst also depends on a woman's genetic predisposition. Younger

women, premenopausal women, and post-menopausal women taking estrogen are likely to have higher hormonal levels and therefore have an increased possibility of having cysts. *(Andolina, p. 158)*

53. **(C)** By the process of elimination, the best choice is that the lesion is a cyst. Although the fibroadenoma, hematoma, and lymph node are all oval or circular lesions, all are of mixed density (radiolucent and radiopaque). *(Tabár, p. 26)*

54. **(B)** Regardless of the kVp, as the kVp increases the relative number of x-rays undergoing Compton interaction also increases. With compression the part is thinner, less kVp is needed to penetrate the part, and therefore there is less Compton scatter. *(Bushong, p. 222)*

55. **(B)** The CBE involves both a visual inspection and palpation of the breast. A visual inspection involves looking for changes in the shape and size and appearance of the breast and nipple while noting any skin dimpling, redness, or swelling. *(ACS, p. 11; Breast Cancer Resource Center: Detection and Symptoms, p. 3)*

56. **(D)** The hypo estimator provides an estimate of the amount of residual hypo in the film in units of grams per square meter. It should be 0.05 g/m² or 5 µg/cm² (micrograms per square centimeter) or less. If the stain indicates that the residual hypo has increased, the test should first be repeated. If the result is the same then the first check should be the water wash tank—it should be full. Water wash flow rates should meet manufacturer's guidelines. The fixer replenishment rate must also be checked, because they too should meet manufacturer's guideline. *(ACR, p. 211)*

57. **(C)** Fibrous and glandular tissue are together described as fibroglandular densities. X-rays pass more easily through fatty tissue than through fibrous or glandular tissue. Fatty areas appear as radiolucent (black or less dense) areas on the mammogram. The fibroglandular tissue is more ra-

diopaque than fatty tissues and results in areas of lower optical density on the mammogram (white or denser areas). *(Andolina, p. 150; Wentz, p. 12)*

58. **(A)** Estrogen and progesterone are two of the many hormones responsible for many physiologic changes in the breast. Estrogen is responsible for ductal proliferation and progesterone for lobular proliferation. Once a woman starts estrogen the changes can be spotty, causing lumps or increased interstitial fluids (cysts) but will generally result in an overall increase in glandular tissue. *(Andolina, p. 149)*

59. **(C)** By process of elimination, the lesion is likely to be a lymph node. Lymph nodes are lesions with mixed density and generally have a radiolucent center corresponding to the hilus. The fibroadenoma, hematoma, and the galactocele are all mixed-density oval or circular lesions, but none has the lucent center typical of the lymph nodes. *(Tabár, pp. 26–28)*

60. **(C)** When comparing the MLO projection to the ML a lateral abnormality will move down on the lateral from its position on the MLO. A medial abnormality will move up on the lateral from its position on the MLO. A centrally located lesion and lesion at the areola will show little or no movement. *(Andolina, p. 260)*

61. **(A)** As the magnification factor increases, to maintain a sharp image the focal spot must be reduced or the thickness of the part has to decrease. The greater the magnification factor, the smaller the focal spot. Small focal spot is therefore used in magnification mammography. Increasing OID increases the magnification factor. *(Andolina, p. 64; Bushong, pp. 264–265)*

62. **(A)** The actual focal spot size is the area on the anode target that is exposed to electrons from the tube current. Because the target is angled, the effective area of the target is made much smaller than the actual area of electron interactions. The effective target is the area projected onto the patient and the

image receptor. The nominal focal spot size is a measure of the effective focal spot size and is the value used when identifying large or small focal spots. *(Bushong, p. 132)*

63. **(A)** Even though men are at a lower risk of developing breast cancer they should be aware of risk factors, especially family history and should report any changes in their breast to a physician. *(ACS, p. 2)*

64. **(D)** The density difference (DD) on the sensitometric control strip is the difference between the average density closest to 2.20 (high density, HD) and the average density closest to but not less than 0.45 (low density, LD). Base plus fog is the density over a clear area of the strip and the mid density (MD) is that closest to 1.20. *(ACR, p. 151)*

65. **(C)** Epithelial hyperplasia is also known as proliferative breast disease and is an overgrowth of cells that line either the ducts or the lobules. When hyperplasia involves the duct it is called ductal hyperplasia or duct epithelial hyperplasia. When it affects the lobules it is referred to as lobular hyperplasia. Depending on how it looks under the microscope it may be classified as usual or atypical. A sebaceous cyst is a pimple-like cyst that occurs in the oil glands of the skin, and the hematoma is a pooling of blood as a result of trauma. Over time a hematoma may calcify, resulting in the formation of an oil cyst. *(Breast Cancer Resource Center: Benign Breast Conditions, p. 7)*

66. **(A)** A ruptured implant shows extracapsular leakage—silicone may leak into the fibrous capsule or may escape from the capsule leaking into the surrounding breast tissues and muscle causing pain or discomfort. In the encapsulated implant the implant hardens or calcifies but does not rupture. A herniated implant shows the implant pushing out of fibrous capsule, but does not indicate a silicone leak. Patients with implant removal may have traces of residual silicone in the breast. *(Andolina, p. 304)*

67. **(C)** The first step is to determine the location of the lesion by applying the rules for lesion movement. When comparing the MLO projection to the ML a lateral abnormality will move down from its position on the MLO. A medial abnormality will move up from its position on the MLO. A centrally located lesion and lesions at the areola will show little or no movement. Once the location of the lesion is determined, an XCCL for a lateral lesion or the CV for medial lesions will locate the lesion in the CC position. The AX images the axilla of the breast only and is not needed. *(Andolina, p. 265)*

68. **(A)** During ductography, a collecting duct that ends at the nipple is cannulated and a small amount of contrast is injected. Generally, 1–5 cc of contrast is enough to fill the duct. *(Andolina, p. 325)*

69. **(C)** The glandular dose is used in mammography because the biological effects of radiation are most likely to be related to the total energy absorbed by glandular tissue. The glandular dose is the average radiation dose to the glandular tissue in the middle of the breast. The other measure of dose is the entrance skin exposure (ESE). The ESE is most often referred to as the patient dose. It is the exposure at the skin's surface. In mammography the ESE may be very high because of low-energy x-rays but the dose falls quickly as the x-rays penetrate the breast. *(Bushong, p. 553)*

70. **(C)** Obtaining a magnified image requires that the OID be increased while maintaining a constant SID. Any change in OID will result in a corresponding change in SOD. To maintain a sharp image, a small focal spot must be used in magnification. *(Bushong, p. 303)*

71. **(D)** QC testing should always be performed by the dedicated quality control personnel or the same individual. Here the mammographer would be the most obvious person. *(ACR, p. 90; Andolina, p. 118)*

72. **(B)** Galactoceles are small, milk-filled cysts with a high fat content. They are associated with lactation, may be mixed density, and are circular–oval with sharply defined contours. A hematoma is associated with breast trauma

and the oil cyst appears mammographically as shell-like calcifications. Lymph nodes typically have a central radiolucent area corresponding to the hilus. *(Tabár, pp. 26–29)*

73. **(A)** During pregnancy and lactation, breast density increases due to physiologic changes, milk production, and increased blood supply. The changes are a result of the action of estrogen, progesterone, and prolactin, which cause a proliferation of the ductal and lobular structure of the breast and an increase in blood flow. *(Andolina, pp. 146–152)*

74. **(C)** Most glandular tissue is found centrally and extends laterally toward the axilla in the upper outer quadrant. This distribution increases or decreases with hormonal fluctuations, but generally mirrors the opposite breast. *(Andolina, p. 142; Wentz, p. 13)*

75. **(C)** Mammography uses very-low-energy kVp and it is very important that the x-ray tube window not attenuate the low-energy photons. Most mammography units have either borosilicate or beryllium windows. The low atomic number of these materials allows an inherent filtration of approximately 0.1 mm Al. The material of the glass window has no effect of scattered radiation, nor can it increase or decrease the output of the x-ray tube. *(Bushong, p. 312; Wentz, p. 18)*

76. **(C)** Compression is important in mammography to reduce breast thickness, radiation dose, and motion unsharpness. Compression also separates superimposed areas of the breast tissue and brings abnormalities closer to the image receptor. Unfortunately, compression is painful for some women. In general, the breast should be compressed until taut to ensure adequate compression. Compression, however, should not be applied to cause the patient severe pain. *(Andolina, p. 58)*

77. **(C)** The greater the magnification factor the greater the skin dose to the patient. In magnification the patient dose increases because the breast is closer to the source and because additional exposure is required because of reciprocity law failure. The small focal spot size used to

maintain a sharp image requires that the mA be reduced with a corresponding increase in exposure time. *(Andolina, p. 185; Carlton, p. 582)*

78. **(B)** The actual focal spot size is the area on the anode target that is exposed to electrons from the tube current. As the size of the focal spot decreases, the heating of the target is concentrated into a smaller area. In the design known as the line focus principle, the target is angled allowing a larger area for heating while maintaining a small effective focal spot. Because the target is angled the effective area of the target is made much smaller than the actual area of electron interactions. The effective target is the area projected onto the patient and the image receptor. As the target angle is made smaller the effective focal spot decreases (Figure 7–8). *(Bushong, p. 131)*

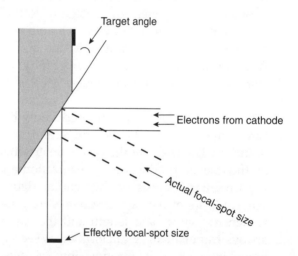

Figure 7–8. Line focus principle. As the size of the focal spot decreases, the heating of the target concentrates into a smaller area. Angling the target makes the effective focal spot size much smaller than the actual focal spot size. This line focus principle allows a large area for heating while keeping the effective focal spot small. Decreasing the target angle causes a corresponding decrease in effective focal spot size.

79. **(D)** Sterostatic localization and needle localization are both reserved for nonpalpable lesions. Ductography outlines the ductal system and is indicated if the patient has nipple discharge. If the lesion is palpable and highly suspicious for malignancy, the next step is a core or surgical biopsy. Ultrasound could also be used to evaluate masses to determine whether they are solid or cystic. *(Andolina, p. 314; Wentz, pp. 87–89)*

80. (B) The patient's face should be turned away from the side under examination curving the neck and head around the face shield. This ensures that medial tissue can be pulled onto the image receptor. This is important because eliminating medial breast tissue from the CC projection may eliminate this tissue from the study. *(Andolina, p.188; Wentz, pp. 58–60)*

81. (A) In the XCCL and the CC the central rays are directed superiorly to inferiorly; therefore, 12 o'clock and 6 o'clock lesions will be superimposed. The AT images the axilla and would miss any 6 o'clock lesion. In the MLO, the beam is directed medially to laterally separating the upper aspect of the breast (12 o'clock position) from the lower aspect (6 o'clock position). *(Andolina, p. 198; Wentz, p. 60)*

82. (C) This represents the standard terminology adopted by the American College of Radiology (ACR). The Cleopatra view is an old term given to a projection similar to the current AX. All projections in mammography are compression or compressed views. *(ACR, p. 24)*

83. (D) Casting calcifications are produced when carcinoma in situ fills the ducts and their branches. The shape of the cast is determined by the uneven production of calcification and the irregular necrosis of the cellular debris. The contours of the cast are always irregular in density, width, and length and the cast is always fragmented. A calcification is seen as branching when it extends into adjacent ducts. Additionally, the width of the ducts determines the width of the castings. Eggshell-like and needle-like, sharply outlined, or elongated branching calcifications are typically benign mammographically. Granulated sugar or crushed stone calcifications are called granular-type calcifications and are mammographically malignant. *(Tabár, pp. 150, 208)*

84. (B) From the nipple orifice, a connecting duct immediately widens into the lactiferous sinus or ampulla. The ampulla is a pouch-like structure that holds milk (when it is being produced). These ducts branch into smaller and smaller ducts until becoming a lobule. The

lobule is also called the terminal ductal lobular unit (TDLU) and holds the milk-producing elements of the breast. *(Logan-Young, p. 15)*

85. (D) The nipple cannot always be imaged in profile because some women will not have a centrally located nipple. (It will either be in the top half or bottom half of the breast.) In such situations imaging the nipple in profile will actually lose posterior breast tissue. Additional views of the nipple area are only necessary if the nipple looks like a lesion, the woman has a nipple or retroareolar abnormality (such as nipple discharge or a lesion), for proper measurement in preoperative localizations, or if the patient is male. Male patients have rudimentary breast buds lying directly behind the nipple. Only by placing the nipple in profile will this area be visualized clearly. *(Andolina, p. 182)*

86. (C) The AT projection best demonstrates the axillary tail of the breast. The medial and subareolar areas are not visualized on the AT projection. The lower inner quadrant describes the medial portion of the breast. *(Andolina, p. 230; Wentz, p. 66)*

87. (C) In this case the patient's chin was not elevated for the MLO projection. Pressure on the film after the exposure causes plus-density artifacts. This is inconsistent with malposition of the mirror, which would cause a rectangular-shaped artifact in the center of the film. The other alternative, the patient's shoulder, would only be imaged if the entire axilla were also imaged. *(Andolina, p. 104)*

88. (B) A hematoma is associated with breast trauma. Galactoceles are small, milk-filled cysts with a high fat content associated with lactation. Fibroadenomas are benign tumors common in women at any age and the intramammary lymph nodes can be found in any quadrant of the breast and are not related to injury. *(Andolina, p. 165; Tabár, p. 26)*

89. (D) Patients have breast tissue ranging from fatty to thicker, more glandular tissue. Adequate penetration of the glandular tissue depends on the kVp selection. In mammography, the use of single emulsion films with single-backed screens is necessary to enhance contrast, but results in a relatively higher patient dose. Dose in mammography is kept low because of the inherent soft tissue structure of the breast. Viewing conditions should not determine the exposure selection, but the target material determines the energy of the x-ray beam produced. *(Wentz, p. 46)*

90. **(B)** Generally when the shoulders are not relaxed or if the height of the image receptor is too high most of the axilla and shoulders will fall into the compression area. The thick area of the axilla and shoulder will cause the compression paddle to stop at maximum without adequate compression being applied to the lower breast (nipple area). *(Andolina, p. 198; Wentz, p. 79)*

91. **(C)** Ultrasound does not image microcalcifications well. The TAN projection is useful in assessing skin calcification and the spot compression view increases compression over a specific area to eliminate pseudomasses. Magnification, however, magnifies the area of interest allowing the number, distribution, and type of calcifications to be clearly seen. *(ACR, pp. 59–60)*

92. **(A)** Paget's disease of the breast (first described by Jean Paget in 1874) is a special form of ductal carcinoma associated with eczematous changes of the nipple. Generally it presents as a malignant nipple lesion. *(Tabár, p. 190)*

93. **(D)** The rolled views are helpful when dense breast tissue is superimposed on a lesion. The dense tissue is rolled off the lesion. *(ACR, p. 67; Wentz, p. 68)*

94. **(D)** The specimen must be imaged after biopsy to ensure that the lesion was completely removed. In imaging the specimen it should be compressed and magnified to prevent the appearance of pseudomasses and to assess calcifications. The specimen should also be compared to the initial mammogram

films. Imaging the specimen before the surgery is completed will allow the surgeon to take an additional biopsy specimen if indicated. *(Andolina, p. 320)*

95. **(C)** The LMO is useful for patients with prior chest surgery or patients with pacemakers, which prevent compression to the medial breast. The LMO is an inferolateral to superomedial projection. The x-ray tube is angled approximately 125° (Figure 7–9). The image receptor is positioned at the medial aspect of the breast and compression is applied from the lateral aspect. *(Andolina, p. 217; Wentz, p. 70)*

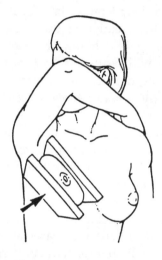

Figure 7–9.   (© 2000 The American Registry of Radiologic Technologists.)

96. **(B)** The actual focal spot size is the area on the anode target that is exposed to electrons from the tube current. Because the target is angled, the effective area of the target is made much smaller than the actual area of electron interactions. The effective target is the area projected onto the patient and the image receptor. The nominal focal spot size is a measure of the effective focal spot size and is the value used when identifying large or small focal spots. *(Bushong, p. 132)*

97. **(D)** Radiation and surgical treatment will cause changes in the breast and can cause calcium formation. Although the rate of recurrence after lumpectomy is relatively low,

magnification views of the tumor bed should be compared with radiographs taken after surgery but *before* radiation treatment. *(Andolina, p. 260)*

98. **(C)** The ML is useful in determining whether a lesion is medially or laterally located. If the MLO projection is compared to the ML, a medial lesion will move up from its position on the MLO. A lateral lesion will move down from its position on the MLO. A lesion that is centrally located will show little or no movement. *(Andolina, p. 265)*

99. **(D)** Films should be processed promptly because of latent image fading. If the time between the creation of the latent image and processing is 8 hours or more, the biggest change will be in loss of film speed. However, both density and contrast will also decrease. *(ACR, p. 132; Andolina, p. 85)*

100. **(A)** All three methods can be used to minimize scattered radiation in general radiography. The higher the kVp the higher the level of scattered radiation. Reducing the thickness of the part will allow a reduction in kVp, hence, a reduction in scattered radiation. Scattered radiation increases as the field size increases; therefore, reducing the field size will reduce the amount of scattered radiation. Unfortunately, reducing the field size is not an option in mammography. Mammography units have only two available field sizes, regardless of breast size. *(Bushong, p. 223)*

101. **(B)** The MQSA was established on October 27, 1992 to establish minimum national standards for mammography. Under the MQSA requirements, the FDA can authorize individual states to certify mammography facilities, conduct inspections, and enforce the MQSA quality standards. After October 1994, the MQSA required all legal providers of mammography services to be accredited by an approved accreditation body and certified by the FDA. The FDA cannot ensure that all women have access to a certified mammography facility. *(Accreditation and Certification Overview)*

102. **(D)** The MQSA final regulations require facilities to have a written and documented policy of resolving consumer complaints. The facility may select its own format. Medical outcome audit is required by MQSA to follow up positive mammographic assessments and to correlate pathology results with the radiologist's findings. Record keeping refers to the section of MQSA standards dealing with the maintenance of mammography films and reports in a permanent file (for not less than 5 years, or not less than 10 years if no additional mammograms of the patient are performed at the facility, or longer if required by state or local laws). To satisfy the communication-of-results section of the standards, all mammographic facilities must send each patient a summary of the report, written in lay terms, within 30 days of the mammographic examination. If assessments are suspicious or highly suspicious for malignancy, the facility should contact the patient as soon as possible with the results. *(Accreditation and Certification Overview)*

103. **(B)** A harmartoma is a benign tumor. It is considered self-limiting because the tumor consists of an overgrowth of normal tissue and the tumor cells do not reproduce. Breast lesions associated with trauma and nursing are hematoma and galactocele, respectively. *(Tabár, p. 26; Thomas, p. 836)*

104. **(B)** Parturition is the process of giving birth. In the immature breast a two-layer epithelium of cells lines the ducts and alveoli. After puberty this epithelium proliferates, forming three alveolar cell types—superficial (luminal) A cells, basal B cells (chief cells), and myoepithelial cells. The myoepithelial cells are arranged in a branching, star-like fashion located around the alveoli and excretory milk ducts. Contraction of the myoepithelial cells helps to propel milk toward the nipples. Beneath the epithelium is connective tissue that helps to keep the epithelium in place. Between the epithelium and the connective tissue is a layer called the basement membrane. The basement membrane provides support

and acts as a semi-permeable filter under the epithelium. *(Harris, p. 10; Tortora, pp. 105, 1000.)*

105. **(A)** An incomplete finding means that more testing is needed to accurately evaluate the breast. That additional testing can be spot compression or using another modality (for example, ultrasound). The MQSA categories place all mammographic findings in one of the following categories:

- **Negative:** nothing to comment on
- **Benign:** also a negative assessment
- **Probably benign:** finding(s) have a probability of being benign
- **Suspicious:** finding(s) have a definite probability of being malignant
- **Highly suggestive of malignancy:** findings have a high probability of being malignant
- **Incomplete:** when additional imaging evaluation is needed

(Accreditation and Certification Overview)

106. **(D)** Erythema is a redness or inflammation of the skin. Although it can indicate inflammatory breast cancer, it can also be an indication of breast abscess or other infectious changes. Further evaluation and testing, including mammography, would be necessary to determine the cause. *(Tabár, p. 241; Thomas, p. 668)*

107. **(C)** Tamoxifen is a nonsteroidal antiestrogen given to patients with breast cancer. Tamoxifen is considered a palliative treatment because it will not cure the disease but has been proven to reduce the rate of reoccurrence of the tumor and reduce the risk for breast cancer for women at very high risk. The drug can cause serious side effects including an increased risk for endometrial cancer. Radiation therapy may be used to destroy cancer cells remaining after surgery or to reduce the size of a tumor before surgery. Chemotherapy uses a combination of drugs to kill undetected tumor cells that may have migrated to other parts of the body. Antibody therapy works by blocking the effect of the protein HER-2—important in regulating the growth of breast cancer cells. *(ACS, pp. 10–14)*

108. **(D)** Noise on the mammographic film is an undesirable fluctuation in the optical density of the image and will show on the radiographs similar to "snow" on a monitor. The principal cause of radiographic noise is scattered radiation produced by Compton scattering, which reduces contrast. Quantum mottles and film graininess also result in noise on the radiography. Quantum mottle refers to the way x-rays interact with the image receptor. If the image is produced with a few x-ray photons, the quantum mottle will be higher than if the image is produced with many x-ray photons. Film graininess refers to the distribution in size and space of the silver halide grains in the emulsion and is a factor inherent in the image receptor. This factor is not under the control of the mammographer. *(Bushong, p. 254)*

109. **(C)** After puberty the epithelium of the lobules proliferates, becoming multilayered and forming three alveolar cell types, superficial (luminal) A cells, basal B cells (chief cells), and myoepithelial cells. The innermost layer or basal surface of the epithelium consists of myoepithelial cells. Beneath the epithelium is connective tissue that helps to keep the epithelium in place. Between the epithelium and the connective tissue is a layer called the basement membrane. The basement membrane provides support and acts as a semi-permeable filter under the epithelium. *(Tortora, pp. 105, 1000; Harris, p. 10)*

110. **(C)** The "camel's nose" contour refers to the sloping of the breast in the MLO projection due to insufficient compression. The result is poor separation of the breast tissues. Preventing "camel's nose" involves pulling the breast up and out and supporting it during the initial stage of compression. The mammographer should use one hand to maintain support of the breast until enough compression is in place to keep the breast in position. *(ACR, pp. 38–40)*

111. **(C)** The SIO best demonstrates the upper-inner quadrant (UIQ) and the lower-outer quadrant (LOQ) of the breast, free of superimposition. This projection can be used to

demonstrate these quadrants free of the implant using the Eklund compression techniques (Figure 7–10). *(Andolina, p. 208)*

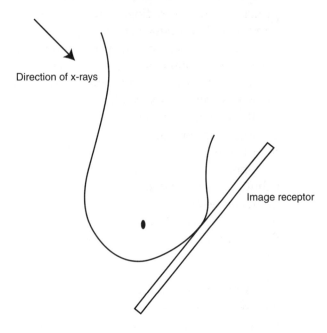

Figure 7–10. In the SIO position the beam is directed from the superior lateral aspect to the inferior medial aspect of the breast.

112. **(D)** The medical audit is used to ensure the reliability of the mammographic image. The interpreting physicians should evaluate all mammographic results for clarity and accuracy at least once every 12 months. The medical audit should also include any cases of breast cancer found after a negative mammography reading. *(Accreditation and Certification Overview: Medical Outcomes Audit Program)*

113. **(B)** The MQSA requires facilities to maintain records to the original mammogram films and report for a period of not less than 5 years and not less than 10 years if no additional mammograms of the patient are performed at the facility. Some state and local laws may require longer storage times. Facilities are also allowed to permanently or temporarily transfer a patient's records to another medical institution, physician, or health care provider if requested by the patient. *(Accreditation and Certification Overview: Record Keeping)*

114. **(B)** Triangulation is used to determine the location of a nonpalpable lesion seen mammographically. One of the purposes of triangulation is to spot compress the lesion for improved separation of breast tissue. Triangulation is also used to determine the shortest skin-to-abnormality distance for the purpose of sterostatic biopsy. To determine the location of the lesion relative to the nipple, the technologist should measure (1) the distance from the nipple to the level of the lesion posteriorly on the CC or MLO projection, (2) from that level to the lesion in the superior-to-inferior (as on the MLO) or medial-to-lateral direction (as on the CC), and (3) from the lesion to the skin surface (Figure 7–11). *(ACR, p. 56)*

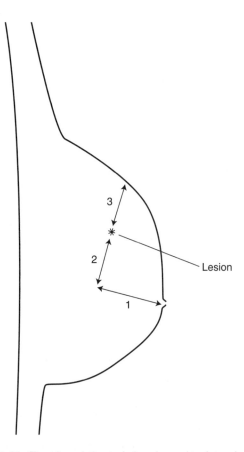

Figure 7–11. The triangulation technique is used to determine the shortest skin-to-abnormality distance in the MLO projection. **1** = distance from nipple to the level of the lesion posteriorly. **2** = distance from level to lesion. **3** = distance from lesion to skin surface.

115. **(D)** Peau d' orange describes the skin of the breast wherein the breast skin thickens and resembles an orange. The condition occurs secondary to obstruction of the axillary lymphatic and may be a result of either benign or malignant conditions such as inflammatory carcinoma. Plasma cell mastitis or ductal ectasia are both inflammatory conditions. Ductal ectasia involve the lactiferous ducts and may or may not cause nipple discharge or inversion. Both conditions are characterized by the presence of plasma cells surrounding a dilated duct. *(Tabár, pp. 199, 203; Thomas, p. 582)*

Index

Pages followed by f indicate figure.

A

AEC. *See* Automatic exposure control (AEC)
American Cancer Society, breast cancer screening
    guidelines, 5, 9, 111, 124
American College of Radiology, quality control
    tests, 15–17
Anechoic, 81
Artifacts, 50
Aspiration, fine needle, 67, 74, 79, 106
Automatic exposure control (AEC), 14, 19, 25
    failure of, 19, 25, 87, 100
    placement of detector, 54, 59, 85, 91, 99, 104
Axillary tail (AT) projection, 63, 69–70, 76–77, 100,
    120, 134

B

Beam restriction devices, 14
Beryllium window, 119, 133
Biopsy, core. *See* Core biopsy
Breast
    anatomy of, 35, 39, 41, 44–45, 46, 114, 119, 120,
        122, 127, 134, 137
    blood supply of, 35, 40, 45
    cysts, 116, 130–131
    effects of radiation on, 115, 128–129
    erythema of, 122, 137
    implants. *See* Breast implants
    lymphatic drainage of, 35, 36f, 40, 45
    during pregnancy and lactation, 119, 133
    tissue composition of, 35–36. *See also* Breast tis-
        sue
    of women under age 35, 114, 128
Breast cancer
    classifications of, 1, 5, 8
    diagnostic options, 2, 7, 11
    in males, 113, 117, 127, 132
    mammographic appearance of, 1–2, 36–37, 38f,
        41–42, 41–42f, 47, 47f
    and medical history, 116, 130
    risk factors for, 1, 4, 8, 84, 88–90, 100, 101, 103,
        111, 124
    screening guidelines, 5, 9
    survival rates, 7, 11, 11t, 91, 104
    symptoms of, 4, 8, 84, 98
    treatment options, 2–3
Breast examination. *See* Breast self-examination
    (BSE); Clinical breast examination (CBE)
Breast implants
    mammographic appearance of, 118, 118f, 132
    mammographic technique for, 63, 64–65f, 73,
        78–79, 80f, 86, 89, 100, 103
    types of, 112, 126–127
Breast lesions
    benign, 1, 4, 8, 37, 112, 112f, 125f
    malignant. *See* Breast cancer
Breast self-examination (BSE), 3, 5, 83, 97
    best time for, 115, 129
    frequency of, 6, 9, 113, 128
    methods for, 9–10, 10f, 93, 107
    reasons for, 114, 128
Breast tissue
    fatty, 39, 45, 117, 131
    fibrous, 90, 92, 104, 106
BSE. *See* Breast self-examination (BSE)

C

Calcification(s), 36–37, 42, 47, 90, 90f, 104, 119, 134
Caudocranial projection. *See* From below (FB) pro-
    jection
CBE. *See* Clinical breast examination (CBE)
CC projection. *See* Craniocaudal (CC) projection
Characteristic curve, 20, 27, 27f, 28f, 84, 98, 98f, 114,
    127
Chemotherapy, 2, 5, 9

Cleavage (CV) projection, 63, 86, 100, 119, 134
Clinical breast examination (CBE), 3, 5, 7, 9, 11, 83, 97
    frequency of, 85, 92, 99, 106
    visual inspection during, 117, 131
Coat hanger method, 83, 97
Collimation, 113, 127
    and image quality, 50, 84, 98
Compression, 13–14, 18, 24, 39, 44, 83, 97
    effect on Compton interactions, 117, 131
    and image quality, 50, 54, 59, 87, 92, 101, 106, 112, 126
    importance of, 49, 51–52, 56–57, 85, 99, 120, 135
    level of, 119, 133
    maximum initial, 113, 127
    spot, 66, 73, 91, 92, 105
    test, 17, 22, 30, 118, 132
Compton interactions, 117, 131
Computerized thermal breast imaging, 2
Contrast, 50, 54, 59
Cooper's ligaments, 39, 44, 45, 88, 102, 102f
Core biopsy, 67, 74, 79, 92, 106, 119, 133
Craniocaudal (CC) projection, 61, 62f, 68, 69, 75, 76, 84, 85, 99
    patient position during, 113, 119, 126, 134
Crossover, film, 111, 124, 124f
CV projection. See Cleavage (CV) projection
Cyst(s), 116, 130–131
    aspiration of, 67, 74, 79, 106

D
D log E curve. See Characteristic curve
Darkroom cleanliness, 16
Darkroom fog test, 17, 21, 22, 29–30, 30f
Developer, 90, 91, 104
Digital mammography, 15, 20, 26, 26f, 27f, 92, 105
    H & D curve, 112, 124, 125f
    need for repeat analysis, 114, 128
Distal echo enhancement, 81
Double emulsion systems, 20, 26
Ductal carcinoma, 1, 74, 81
Ductal ectasia, 95, 105, 126
Ductal papilloma, 83, 97, 105
Ductography, 67, 74, 89, 103
    contrast used in, 118, 132

E
Echogenic, 81
Echopenic, 81
Eklund method, 80f
Epithelial hyperplasia, 118, 132

Estrogen replacement therapy, 87, 101
Exaggerated craniocaudal (XCCL) projection, 61, 68, 70, 76, 77, 100
    compression during, 84, 99
Exposure
    control. See Automatic exposure control
    factors, 120, 134
    and image quality, 50, 53, 58

F
False-negatives, 53, 58
FB projection. See From below (FB) projection
Fibroadenoma, 74, 79–81, 104, 126
Film, 15, 19, 26, 84, 98
    crossover, 111, 124, 125f
    effect of damaged, 87, 100
    effect of delayed processing, 121, 136
    for processor quality control, 90, 104
    residual hypo levels in, 117, 131
Filter, 54
    function of, 54, 59
Fine needle aspiration, 67, 74, 79, 106
First-degree relative, 114, 128
Focal spot size, 15, 117, 119, 121, 131–132, 133, 133f, 135
    factors affecting, 19, 25
    for magnification, 90, 104
From below (FB) projection, 63, 91, 93, 105, 107, 115, 128

G
Galactocele, 43, 48, 118, 132
Geometric unsharpness, 57
Grid ratios, 14, 19, 25, 116, 129
Grids. See Mammography grids
Gynecomastia, 88, 92, 102, 105

H
Halo sign, 41, 47
Hamartoma, 122, 136
Heel effect, 18, 24, 24f, 130, 131f
Hematoma, 104, 120, 134
High-contrast imaging, 83, 97
Hormones
    influences on breast tissue, 114, 117, 128, 131
    role in breast cancer, 84, 98, 111, 124
Hurter and Driffield curve. See Characteristic curve
Hyporetention test, 96, 109

I
Image quality, 50
Image receptor, 15

Inframammary crease, 88, 102
Interventional procedures, 67

K
KVp levels
   of mammography units, 13, 18, 24, 88, 101
   selection of, 49, 53–55, 58–60
Kyphosis, 70, 77

L
Labeling, 50, 54, 59
Lactation
   changes in breast during, 119, 133
   mammography during, 40, 41, 46
Lactiferous sinus, 89, 102
Lateromedial (LM) projection, 63
Lateromedial oblique (LMO) projection, 63
Lesions. *See* Breast lesions
Line focus principle, 133f
Lipoma, 43, 48, 91, 104
LM projection. *See* Lateromedial (LM) projection
LMO projection. *See* Lateromedial oblique (LMO) projection
Lobular carcinoma, 1
Localization
   preoperative needle, 67, 74, 79, 96, 110, 113, 126
   stereostatic, 67
   terminology for, 35, 39, 44, 44f
Lumpectomy, 2
   mammography following, 66, 121, 135
Lymph node, 117, 131
Lymphatic drainage, of the breast, 35, 36f, 40, 45

M
Magnetic resonance imaging (MRI), 2, 5, 9
Magnification mammography
   characteristics of, 49, 52–53, 57–58, 72, 78, 83, 92, 118, 132
   contraindications for, 85, 99
   disadvantages of, 87, 101
   uses of, 63, 94, 97, 105, 107, 115, 129
Mammogram
   false-negative, 53, 58
   projections. *See* Projection(s)
Mammography
   accuracy of, 84, 98
   benefits and risks, 3
   digital. *See* Digital mammography
   film for. *See* Film
   of the irradiated breast, 66, 73
   during lactation, 41, 46

magnification. *See* Magnification mammography
   of the male breast, 73, 96, 109
   and mortality reduction, 3
   of patients with difficult body habitus, 66
   of physically impaired patients, 66
   postsurgical, 66, 73, 79, 113, 121, 127, 135
   radiation dose of, 3, 7, 11, 87, 100, 113, 118, 127, 132
   of the small breast, 83, 97, 115, 122, 129, 136
   technical factors in, 49–50
Mammography facility, accreditation, 17, 23, 32, 122, 136
Mammography grids, 14, 19, 25, 89, 93, 103, 107
Mammography Quality Standards Act (MQSA) requirements, 32, 88, 96, 102, 110, 123, 137
Mammography tube, 13, 18, 24, 32, 116, 130f
Mammography units
   design characteristics of, 13
   exposure control, 14
   kVp levels, 13, 18, 24
Mammoplasty, 96, 109
Mastectomy, 2
   mammography following, 66, 73, 79, 113, 127
Medical history, 116, 130
Mediolateral (ML) projection, 63, 94, 107
Mediolateral oblique (MLO) projection, 61, 62f, 68, 69, 71, 75, 76, 86, 86f, 88, 93, 95, 100, 101, 105, 106
   substitute for, 115, 129
Menopause, 41, 46, 84, 98
Microcalcifications, 121, 135
Miraluma imaging, 2
ML projection. *See* Mediolateral (ML) projection
MLO projection. *See* Mediolateral oblique (MLO) projection
Molybdenum, 54, 59, 101
Montgomery's glands, 44, 87, 92, 100, 105
Morgagni's tubules, 39, 44
Multiparity, 46

N
Nipple
   anatomy of, 112, 124
   imaging of, 86, 94, 100, 107, 120, 134
   inverted, 39, 44
Noise, radiographic, 50, 122, 137
Nuclear medicine, 2
Nulliparous, 41, 46

O
Object-to-image receptor distance (OID), 14–15, 112, 117, 126, 131
Oil cyst, 42, 47, 95, 104, 108

P

Pacemaker, 96, 110
Paget's disease, 87, 101, 105, 121, 135
Papilloma, 115, 129
Peau d'orange, 122, 139
Penumbra, 57
Periductal mastitis, 126
Phantom image test, 16, 21, 23, 28–29, 28f, 29f, 32, 34f
    density difference, 87, 100, 114, 127
    objects in, 112, 125, 125f
    requirements for, 115, 128
Photon interaction, 114, 128
Plasma cell mastitis, 126
Pneumocystography, 67, 74, 81
Positron emission tomography (PET), 116, 130
Posterior nipple line (PNL), 68, 75, 75f
Primapara, 46
Processor quality control, 16, 22, 32, 33f, 83, 88, 97, 102
    reestablishing levels of, 114, 127
Projection(s), 61–63, 62f. *See also* Name(s) of specific projection(s)
    comparison of, 68–72, 75–78, 118, 119, 121, 132, 134, 135, 136

Q

Quality control tests, 20–22, 111, 115, 124, 129
    American College of Radiology standards for, 15–17
Quantum mottle, 96, 109, 112, 126

R

Radiation dose. *See* Mammography, radiation dose of
Radiation therapy, 111, 124
Radiographic noise, 50, 122, 137
Reciprocity law, 49
Reject/repeat analysis, 16, 22, 30, 31f, 94, 107
    in digital imaging, 114, 128
    interpretation of, 116, 129
Retromammary space, 84, 99, 116, 130
Rhodium, 54, 58, 88, 101, 102

Rolled projection, 63, 72, 78, 88, 101, 113, 126
    reasons for using, 121, 135

S

Scintigraphy, 2
Screen-cleaning test, 21
Screen/film contact, 17, 30, 30f
Self-examination, breast. *See* Breast self-examination (BSE)
Sensitometer, 16
    density difference on, 118, 132
    testing, 21, 28, 29f
Sensitometric curve. *See* Characteristic curve
Sentinel node mapping, 2
Sharpness, 50, 55, 60
Source-to-image receptor distance (SID), 14
Spatula, 83, 97
Specimen radiography, 67, 73–74, 79
    timing of, 121, 135
Spot compression, 66, 73–74, 79
Spot magnification, 121, 135
Stereostatic localization, 67
System geometry, 14

T

Tail of Spence, 39, 44
Tamoxifen, 122, 137
Tangential (TAN) projection, 63, 68, 70, 76, 77, 83, 97, 98f, 113, 126
Terminal ductal lobular unit (TDLU), 40, 45, 45f
Tissue composition, 35
Triangulation techniques, 123, 138, 138f
Tube, mammography. *See* Mammography tube

U

Ultrasound, 2, 67, 74

W

Wart, 112, 126

X

XCCL projection. *See* Exaggerated craniocaudal (XCCL) projection